D0125437

The Massage Therapist's Handbook

A Practical Guide to the Business of Massage

Michael Alicia

Illustrations by John-Michael Flate

CUYAHOGA COMMUNITY COLLEGE
EASTERN CAMPUS LIBRARY

iUniverse, Inc.
Bloomington

The Massage Therapist's Handbook
A Practical Guide to the Business of Massage

Copyright © 2011 Michael Alicia
Illustrations by John-Michael Flate

All rights reserved. No part of this book may be used or reproduced by
any means, graphic, electronic, or mechanical, including photocopying,
recording, taping or by any information storage retrieval system
without the written permission of the publisher except in the case
of brief quotations embodied in critical articles and reviews.

iUniverse books may be ordered through booksellers or by contacting:

iUniverse
1663 Liberty Drive
Bloomington, IN 47403
www.iuniverse.com
1-800-Authors (1-800-288-4677)

Because of the dynamic nature of the Internet, any Web addresses or
links contained in this book may have changed since publication and
may no longer be valid. The views expressed in this work are solely those
of the author and do not necessarily reflect the views of the publisher,
and the publisher hereby disclaims any responsibility for them.

Any people depicted in stock imagery provided by Thinkstock are models,
and such images are being used for illustrative purposes only.

Certain stock imagery © Thinkstock.

ISBN: 978-1-4620-0426-3 (pbk)
ISBN: 978-1-4620-0427-0 (ebk)

Printed in the United States of America

iUniverse rev. date: 8/12/2011

*To Robert Calhoun for his unending faith and encouragement,
Steven Cantor for his support and advice, and mostly to Kate Edgar
for her professional expertise and tireless editorial handiwork.*

Contents

Introduction

When Bill Clinton was campaigning for president in 1992, he tried to stay focused on what he thought was most important to the voters in order to get elected. His now-famous sound bite, "It's the economy, stupid," caught my attention. At the time, I was embarking on my new massage career, and I adopted a similar phrase for myself, "It's about the work, stupid," to help me stay focused on what I still believe to be the most important aspect for a successful career in massage. Since then, I have hijacked another phrase and turned it into a creed: "If the work is good, they will come." So with these two phrases, you know the basic premise of this book. I firmly believe that if our work is good and informed and focused and compassionate, supported by nothing but the best intentions, success will surely follow.

These make for terrific catchphrases, but of course there are many more practical considerations for establishing a successful practice in massage. For the beginning therapist navigating through this array of business decisions, from what to practice to where to practice, from what to charge to when to work, it can be truly daunting, if not frightening. A massage therapist is not unlike a performer leaving school for a career in music or show business. Both have been taught their crafts, but with scant attention paid to actually getting work or running a business. Developing the artist in us and working on our craft is fundamental to success, but we must also learn ways to develop and maintain our business. Some therapists do not want to spend time and energy worrying about business decisions and so choose to work for others in spas or doctor's offices. This is a perfectly legitimate career choice and serves its purpose for the therapist and for the community. But even when working for someone else, we need to be aware of the practical aspects of a career in massage therapy.

This book aims to provide the beginning therapist with the tools to start, develop, and maintain a successful massage practice. The quotes sprinkled throughout the text are from friends and colleagues in the massage profession whom I have interviewed over the years. All of them gave generously of their time and experience to reflect on the issues that have confronted them in their own massage practices and the qualities that have contributed to their success.

I hope that *The Massage Therapist's Handbook* will help you launch a successful and rewarding practice of your own.

Acknowledgments

My initial intention for this book was to collect a series of interviews with successful massage therapists from around the country, discussing their paths to success. I developed an outline whereby we would talk about the quality of their training and then their initial foray into the business of massage. I wanted to hear how, once they left school, they established their practices and what advice they could impart to the beginning therapist to shed some light on the practical real-world way of getting started in the profession. I traveled around the country collecting interviews only to discover in the end that the material did not have a cohesive element that connected all of this valuable information. I also recognized that the interviews had a lot in common, not only with my experience and way of thinking but also with each other. Only then did I realize that I needed to write my opinions of how to start a successful practice and support my ideas with the interviews. Following is a list of contributors to the book in the form of quotations interspersed throughout the text.

Diane graduated from the Swedish Institute in New York City in 1990. She started her massage career working with professional track-and-field athletes, which eventually led to her working with the athletes at the Summer Olympics in Barcelona. She worked as a therapist at the renowned Canyon Ranch spa in Tucson, Arizona, where her background in business led to a managerial position. She parlayed her experience there into a career that focused more on spa business development and training with the intention of raising the overall standard of the massage business. Working again with Canyon Ranch, she helped develop and open spas around the country and even on the Queen Mary II, where she was responsible for training and development. She currently works for Cortiva, a company that owns several massage schools across the country, where she works to raise the overall standard of massage education.

Peggy is a fifty-seven-year-old woman who lives and works in Melbourne, Florida. She started practicing as a massage therapist before becoming a Rolfer (structural integrationist), almost eleven years ago. She worked for a brief time as a psychotherapist before getting involved with bodywork, which helped her integrate her work into a more Eastern form of bodywork, incorporating balancing the body, the mind, and the spirit. She especially enjoys working with trauma patients.

Denise is forty-one years old and practices massage in San Francisco and Sonoma County. She has been in practice for thirteen years and opened a second office five years ago. She has what she calls a Somatic practice, which is therapeutic massage that incorporates energy and movement work in addition to body-based counseling.

Barry is a forty-eight-year-old reverend-turned-bodyworker who lives in Santa Monica, California. He has been "laying hands" on people since 1988. He started by studying Shiatsu before incorporating energy medicine, therapeutic massage, and structural integration into his practice. He has two offices, one in Santa Monica and one in Culver City, in addition to making house calls.

Robert is forty-four years old and lives in Miami Beach, Florida, and first studied massage at the University of Florida in the '70s. His professional massage career began in 1989 after graduating from Educating Hands, a well-known massage school in Miami. He practices Swedish, deep tissue, neuromuscular, Trager, and Thai massage. He worked as a therapist for the '95 Special Olympics and the '96 Olympic Games in Atlanta.

Tamara lives in Chicago and is thirty-one years old and has practiced massage for four and a half years. She graduated from the Chicago School of Massage Therapy. She first started practicing as a therapist at the Chicago Board of Trade before partnering with another therapist and opening a storefront where they employ two other therapists.

Tony is thirty-five years old and lives in Denver, Colorado. He graduated from the Massage Therapy Institute of Colorado in Denver. He started his massage career working with a hotel massage service before doing spa work and corporate chair massage. He now earns most of his massage income from private clients with the occasional hotel client. He supplements his income with a part-time job in the corporate sector where he solicits massage clients for his private practice.

Theresa graduated from the Swedish Institute in New York City in 1995 and became licensed there in '96. She started her massage career working nights, five to six shifts a week, for a company that provides massage services to gyms in New York, while also maintaining a full-time secretarial day job. After nine months she quit her day job and struck out on her own to develop a private practice while maintaining her gym job. Eventually she developed her private practice so she could leave her gym job. After the events of September 11, she relocated to Seattle, where she has carved out a niche doing house calls and opened her own private office space.

Mary is a graduate of the Swedish Institute in New York City, where she established a successful practice before moving to Amherst, a small town in Massachusetts. Establishing a successful practice in a small town was both a challenge and an adventure and ultimately proved rewarding both personally and professionally.

Alexis is fifty-five years old and graduated from the Swedish Institute in New York City in 1983. She has also been a teacher of massage at the Swedish Institute for sixteen years and at various other schools around the country. In addition to teaching, she has a full-time practice at her home on Long Island, where she works with terminally ill clients as well as the well-heeled transient summer crowd.

1. The Four-Step Guide for Success

"There are no secrets to success. It's the result of preparation, hard work, and learning from failure."

—Colin Powell

The Four-Step Guide for Success

Remember: It's about the work!

1. Continue your education
    Workshops
    Exchanges
    Receive massage

2. Get a job (in a spa, gym, or doctor's office)
    Practice your craft
            Evaluation skills
            Body mechanics
            Build strength and stamina
            Learn new techniques

3. Create a business plan
    Make decisions; visualize goals
    Formulate a plan
            Short- and long-term goals
            Outline individual steps

4. Network
    Sell yourself
    Distribute business cards
    Talk about massage
    Join professional or social organizations
    Explore related bodywork businesses in your area

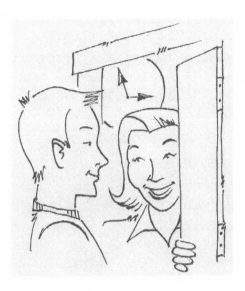

Golden Rule 1

Dependability and punctuality confer credibility.

Success, it is said, is mostly about showing up.
Show up. On time. And do what you say you will.
McDonald's is successful because people know what to expect.

2. Qualities for Success

To determine the essential qualities and characteristics one needs to be a successful massage therapist, I conferred with my colleagues at the Swedish Institute in New York City, where I have been a teacher since 1994. We distilled the vast array of talents and characteristics down to four basic qualities:

Talent
People Skills
Business Skills
Discipline

Talent and good work are the foundations of a successful business. People skills involve good communication skills and, mostly, listening. Business skills include PR, marketing, and selling yourself. Discipline involves body maintenance, continuing education, and simple day-to-day operational skills, like returning phone calls promptly and showing up on time. These are the basic tools that are necessary to build a successful practice in massage.

Talent

Talent is subjective. What one person perceives as creative and innovative may seem ordinary and mundane to another. Talent can also be defined as instinct or even as intuition. It is one of the nebulous qualities we possess that make us unique.

Any art form requires a certain degree of talent, instinct, and intuition. Exactly how a photographer knows when to press the shutter to capture an inspiring moment or how a painter chooses the perfect color to elicit

8

an emotional response is inexplicable. Of course, each of these artists must also study the technical aspects of their crafts, but it is individual experience, values, and passion that make their work unique and could be defined as inspiration, the key ingredient for developing talent. We might add to that a curious mind. If the impetus for practicing massage revolves around, for example, making money, I suspect that the work will not be all that inspired or client-centered. However, if the work is client-centered, supported by a strong desire to be beneficial along with a thirst for knowledge, the quality of the work will grow, and the client's impression is sure to be affected positively. High-quality training coupled with a strong desire to be good and effective is the prerequisite for developing whatever talent we may innately possess.

Some people will like our work and some won't. No one therapist can be everybody's cup of tea. Knowing this will help our artist's ego when our work is not appreciated. I firmly believe that there is room for all of us to be successful. When it seems that our colleagues are getting more clients or our phones are not ringing, rather than begrudging others' success or belittling our own talents, we should take a deep, nurturing breath, reaffirm our commitment to the work, and acknowledge that the universe provides for us when we are ready. In the meantime, there is always room to adapt and fine-tune your work: "Work on the work." Start by evaluating your work as objectively as you can; then ask for feedback from friends and colleagues whose opinions you trust and value. Remember, it's all about the work.

> I think people who succeed in this field simply *are* massage therapists, either by natural talent or through hard work and craft. Whether you succeed financially, however, depends on whether you learn to be a businessperson, your luck, and your timing; and that's a whole different kettle of fish.
>
> Theresa, Seattle, WA

People Skills: First and Foremost, Listening

I can't overemphasize the value of listening in our profession. Listening informs our work from the first interaction through the first meeting, the evaluation and intake, the initial touch of the session, and even in the follow-up after the session. We are listening with our whole being: our ears, our hands, and even our intuition. Remember, we are in the health-care profession. People know that we care by the way we listen. We should let our work do our speaking for us.

> It comes down to the core issue of really working and knowing who you are. The people who succeed are the kind of people who can be personable and essentially let it be about the other person.
>
> Denise, San Francisco, CA

Smiling is another very simple people skill to cultivate. This idea may seem simplistic and even silly, but it is amazing how many therapists in the day-to-day grind of work forget to be friendly. People are attracted to friendly people. Tired, worried, sad, complaining, chatty, and needy people are a turn-off. Many successful service-industry professions spend time and money helping employees develop their people skills. In the restaurant business, "the customer is always right" for a reason: the customer has the money and the option to go somewhere else. Smiling and saying, "Hello," "How are you," "Have a nice day," "Thank you," "Excuse me," "I'm sorry," "You're right," "Let me get that for you," "How are you feeling?" "Are you comfortable?" "Can I get you anything?" "Cold water?" "Hot tea?" "Warm blanket?" "Soft pillow?" "Can I help you?" "With your coat?" "To the elevator?" "Down the stairs?" "With your packages?" "To your car?" or any of a multitude of polite gestures are the simple bedrock to developing a long-lasting relationship with our clients.

Communicating articulately, professionally, and with empathy and compassion is a vital skill to foster. Many people are completely ignorant about how their bodies work or even what they do to make their bodies hurt. The ability to explain in a simple and concise way what we believe and what our intention is for our session with them is an invaluable tool for success. Regardless of our professional assessment, we should come to it only after listening and acknowledging our client's experience and point of view. Compassion is best exhibited through listening. Even the most out-of-touch client has the first-hand experience we need to inform our decisions. It's important to have a point of view and a clear intention, but not as important as hearing and honoring our client's point of view. We don't have to agree with their points of view, but we have to hear them and acknowledge them before explaining our intention. Even if our clients don't want to be involved in the session, they want to be heard and acknowledged, first and foremost, and then informed. Simple is better. If they want more information, they will ask.

> I think that's the key, if we'd only listen to the whispers when they come in. That's really the thing that makes the difference, all the difference in the world. My thing is to let my ego fall back out of the way to just be there for them, with them, because it has nothing to do with me, it has everything to do with them—who they are, why they're there, and how I can serve them.
>
> Barry, Los Angeles, CA

Business Skills: Developing an Ongoing Relationship

Business is about selling. If we asked a spa owner what he was selling, he would probably say he was selling time. He has rooms with therapists, and he is selling hour-long time slots for the therapists to do massage. From the therapist's point of view, though, the product is a relationship. We are trying to develop an ongoing relationship where we provide massage. I think all business is about developing relationships: with the customer and the community, with colleagues and related businesses.

Essentially, then, we are selling ourselves. From a business point of view, our product is us. We embody our work. Our education, our talent, our personality, our physicality, our history, our ability to communicate, and our empathy all inform our clients about the work they will receive and how they will receive it. If the work is good but the package is unappealing, the relationship will end. There are good and bad ways of selling oneself. An aggressive sell is not a particularly good approach in the world of massage. Good work is our greatest selling point. If the work is good, people will tell other people and business will grow.

Another proactive and subtle way to sell ourselves is to practice what we preach. I constantly tell my students that if they become successful in the world of massage, their lifestyles will change. If they truly embody the new vocabulary they are learning, their lives can't help but change. If our work is congruent with our lifestyle, people will recognize that we speak from experience and will trust our opinions. Lasting and healthy relationships are built on trust.

Another aspect of our relationship with our clients is education. Remember, simple is better. Helping our clients recognize their bad habits and offering *simple* alternatives without sounding condescending or preachy helps them learn how to help themselves. (I'm speaking about suggestions that fall within our scope of practice, of course. Why their new hair color is all wrong for their eyes, we'll leave to their hairdresser.) If we educate our clients and empower them to take charge of their physical well-being, we help nurture a trusting and long-lasting relationship.

Being conversant with anatomy and physiology and even the history of the profession makes us sound professional and well educated. The ability to answer questions like "What muscle is that?" or "Does Swedish massage come from Sweden?" simply and conversationally can not only educate our clients but can impress them as well.

Starting and growing a business requires marketing and even public relations skills, which I will cover in depth in chapter 7. There are whole companies and career paths dedicated to these skills and professions, and they are important. But one of the things I love most about massage is the individual relationship I have with each of my clients. No amount of market analysis or demographic studies will provide for the success of a massage practice like simply focusing on the one-on-one relationship with the client. Once we have built a solid core of clients, they become our best PR and marketing department.

A successful business is built one client, one massage, one relationship at a time.

Discipline: A Regular Focus

The word "discipline" is both a noun and a verb and has several connotations with regard to the field of massage. The roots of massage stretch back millennia, to China over 4,500 years ago, where medicine and bodywork were inextricably tied to the martial arts. There were different schools and disciplines that practiced different physical and mental techniques to focus the energy in the body. These techniques were used to promote balance and healing as well as for self-defense, and they required the discipline, or mental and physical self-control, to perceive and cultivate *qi*, or energy. Discipline implies that energy is focused regularly toward a particular goal.

Massage, like the martial arts, is a living art and therefore requires the discipline of practice. Massage therapists, like doctors, are said to "have a practice" because our craft, like the bodies we work on, is vital, changeable, and malleable and thus requires constant attention. The demands and rigors of practicing massage are varied and extensive. Having the physical strength and sensitivity along with the emotional reserve and the mental intuition to do the work in a professional, knowledgeable, and empathetic way all require the investment of time and energy. Focusing and developing the body, the mind, and the spirit in concert is the discipline that is massage. There are no shortcuts. The successful massage therapist finds that the discipline of practicing massage often involves a lifestyle change. Using one's body to make money requires a tremendous investment in time. Developing the mind and the spirit (small words but huge ideas) accentuates for the aspiring therapist the enormity of the discipline required to be successful and effective in the field of massage.

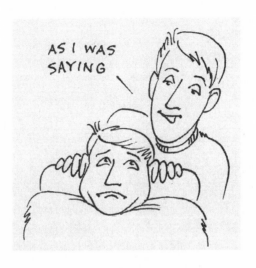

Golden Rule 2

Massage therapists are meant to be felt, not heard.

Keep your problems to yourself.
Some people like to talk; many don't.
Know the difference.

3. Why Massage? Know Thyself

As part of the application process to the Swedish Institute, an aspiring student must write an essay on having received both a Swedish massage and a shiatsu treatment (since the program includes both modalities). It's always shocking to me to see the number of applicants who have never received a massage of any kind before. That seems to me to be like an aspiring athlete having never played the sport. How on earth do these students know that they will like doing or even receiving massage? One of the first things I want my beginning students to think about is why they want to become a massage therapist. On a first meet-and-greet session with beginning students, easily the most common response is, "I want to help people." That is certainly a noble aspiration, but it is not enough.

> If you choose to be a massage therapist, it would be helpful and skillful if you asked yourself, "Why am I choosing to do this? Am I choosing to do this because it's something that makes a contribution in the world?" If it's something that adds value for the people that you're working with and for yourself, then that's a good day and you're doing this for the right reasons. If making a lot of money is what you want, then you really don't want to do bodywork. It's hard work, and if you want to do it to make money, go sell pharmaceuticals; you can make a lot more money.
>
> Barry, Los Angeles, CA

Another common response—"I want to be a healer"—needs reexamining, because I believe we are "healers" to ourselves only. A better word to explain our intention might be "facilitator." As therapists, we facilitate other people healing themselves. This may seem like a

18

semantic play on words, but it is, I think, the foundation of what needs to be client-centered work. We can never completely separate ourselves from our ego (to do so would be to separate ourselves from the artist, the instinct, and the inspiration that informs our work). But, by definition, client-centered means we need to set our ego, our needs, aside and put those of our clients first.

Other reasons for choosing a career in massage therapy might include:
"I want to make a difference."
"I want to change careers."
"I want a part-time job."
"I need a hobby."
"I'm naturally a caretaker."
"People say I'm good at it."

None of these reasons are bad, at least initially.

After getting to know students a little better, though, I start to wonder if some of their reasons for pursuing a career in massage therapy are more like:
"I want to be admired."
"I want to be in charge."
"I'm a control freak."
"I like the power differential."
"I want to be an authority figure."
"I want to meet girls."
"I want to see people naked."
"I want to make a lot of money."
"How hard can it be?"

Above all, I challenge my new students to be honest with themselves about what they want and what they expect from a career in massage. Invariably, when students become more aware of the commitment and dedication required to become a healthy therapist, their intentions change—hopefully, for the better.

Only hours of dedicated and disciplined training and practice can prepare a massage therapist for the work required, whether it is full-time or part-time.

> It's not about money. People think, *Oh, I can make a hundred dollars an hour.* It's a very hard way to make a hundred dollars.
>
> Peggy, Melbourne, FL

> There is this belief that you're going to come out of school and work on your own and really make good money. And you can. But you have to know how to manage and be organized. Only a certain percentage of people can really pursue that successfully.
>
> Diane, New York, NY

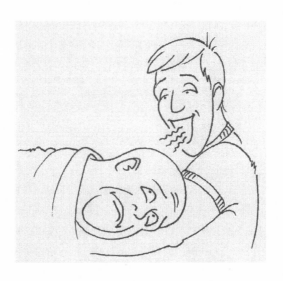

Golden Rule 3

Bad breath is bad for business.

For Buddha's sake, rethink garlic, onions, cigarettes, and perfume.
PS: Wear deodorant!

4. Education

Formal Training

Focusing on "the work" is a recurring theme in this book. When I talk about "the work," I am essentially speaking about education. Whether through formal education, continuing education, or even a single massage session, we are practicing how to be better massage therapists. Our education never ends. We are said to "practice" massage because we are constantly shaping, adapting, and learning in order to suit the individual needs of our clients. The artist studies with different teachers, practicing different styles and using different mediums to develop his own style. The scientist starts her education, learning how to think and formulate ideas, by first acquiring a broad background before focusing on a chosen field. Massage therapy is both an art and a science, and it requires a never-ending educational process in order to stay scientifically current and artistically vital.

There are diverse formal educational programs across the country predicated upon the requirements of individual states or cities. Therefore a recent graduate embarking on a new career as a massage therapist will be better equipped with a formal education that is comprehensive and diverse in its approach. Such a curriculum may be heavy in science classes like anatomy, physiology, and pathology to begin with but also includes the more ethereal energetic arts like shiatsu, Reiki, or reflexology. This will give the beginning practitioner a well-rounded starting point from which to begin the exploration and practice of massage.

Massage is fast becoming a readily accepted form of complementary health care both in the medical community and in the general population. Massage programs across the country are graduating highly trained therapists eager to learn and fill a therapeutic void the medical establishment has spurned for years. The general public is experiencing and distinguishing good and effective massage therapy and has come to expect it. So in order to be competitive and successful in the field, a massage therapist's skills need to be diverse, well learned, and comprehensive.

As with any educational endeavor, you need to choose a program that addresses your interests and your budget (both time and financial), but you should also weigh these against the program's content and concept. A cursory program may be less expensive and less time consuming but may do little to prepare you (physically, intellectually, and emotionally) for the demanding world of massage therapy.

Before committing to a program of study, try to get statistics on the pass/fail rate of the program's graduates for the area's licensing exam. This will be a clear indication of the program's effectiveness in preparing students for the workplace. You might also ask to audit a class or two to see how the classes are conducted. Talk to current or past students of the program to get feedback on their experiences. Ask them how prepared they felt for doing the work. Did they have the working vocabulary to feel comfortable and confident to do what was expected of them? Were they prepared physically, having been trained adequately in proper body mechanics, in order to provide sustained and effective work without discomfort, pain, or injury? Was any attention paid to developing business skills? Is there a placement or outreach service available for students upon graduation? The educational process never ends, but the foundation upon which we build and grow is vitally important.

Continuing Education

To my graduating students I have often said, "Your education truly begins when your schooling ends." This isn't true literally, but the point I try to make is that they have only just begun to use all the information they have assimilated over the past months or years. Most of what they have learned at this point is merely a shopping list of information in their heads. They need bodies on which to practice and apply this knowledge. They need to work. In Eastern medicine, it is said that one needs the experience of working on a thousand bodies before one hears what the body needs.

Continuing education requirements vary from state to state or, in the case of California, city to city. For the national certification continuing education requirement, check the National Certification Board's website at www.ncbtmb.com. You will also find listings of classes offered by category, by city, and by state.

Continuing education can be as structured and formal as taking a class or as informal as doing an exchange with a colleague. *Each massage you give or get is an extension of your educational process.* When receiving a massage, keep your mind's eye open to how the therapist works. Learning what not to do in a massage can be as valuable as learning a delicious new stroke. Finding a colleague or two with whom you have an affinity, whose work you respect, and with whom you can practice and exchange work and ideas is an invaluable asset and relationship to foster. It is the perfect environment to begin to dissect and practice all the information you have assimilated in your formal education (or recent workshop). In this environment, you get immediate and knowledgeable feedback that will help you begin to develop your own style of work. It also helps to develop a professional relationship that can lead to a referral system or professional network.

> Receiving massage is crucial. For me, it is one of my highest forms of learning and continuing education: to receive massage, to stay connected with what I'm doing with other people.
>
> Denise, San Francisco, CA

> Doing the work and getting worked on is the key. Classroom is only one-tenth; the other nine-tenths is receiving and giving massage.
>
> Barry, Los Angeles, CA

> Continuing education happens from working alongside other
> people and practicing techniques and getting comfortable in the
> field.
>
> Tony, Denver, CO

Each client provides a new canvas for us to practice our art, and every massage we give is an opportunity to learn and experiment. Be careful, however, not to make the client feel like a guinea pig. We need to listen for the subtleties that inform our work and to practice in a confident, comfortable, and assuring manner, but at the same time, always work with newfound inspiration. I challenge my students to constantly explore new ways of working, to keep the work fresh for both them and their clients. We might try something as simple as massaging the arm in a prone position instead of the usual supine approach. When my students have questions, I tell them to "figure it out." This is a phrase that I introduce them to very early in our relationship, and I am always amused at their initial shock at hearing it. I explain that I will always help them to find a way of working, but my intention is to get them to learn how to think and to problem-solve on their own.

Workshops provide a more formal type of continuing education. Listings of classes offered around the country can be found on the websites of the National Certification Board (www.ncbtmb.org) and the AMTA (www.amtamassage.org) and in trade magazines like *Massage Magazine* or *Massage Therapy Journal*. Massage schools, even if they don't offer continuing education themselves, will often have information on other classes available. Some colleges and community colleges offer massage programs and provide a valuable resource for massage-related courses and activities. Massage conventions and trade shows usually offer classes and workshops (and if you plan a vacation around a workshop, you can deduct part of your expenses from your taxes). Conventions and trade shows also provide an excellent opportunity for networking with massage professionals across the country. Getting to know massage therapists in other cities can be a valuable resource for referring your clients who travel.

Often I hear therapists complain that they haven't learned anything new at a workshop. This makes me wonder about their ability to be open to new ideas. I believe if I walk out of a workshop having learned only one new stroke or idea, then it was worth it to me. That one stroke or idea may be the inspiration for a whole new way of working. The workshop environment is also a huge opportunity for building relationships and networking with other therapists. It's a place for exploring what's happening in the profession and staying knowledgeable and current.

> What it actually means to begin to do healing work with people—
> that comes over years of learning how to manage my energy, how
> to take care of myself, and how to manage energetically working
> on someone. I get these from both practicing massage and from
> continuing education.
>
> Denise, San Francisco, CA

So when I speak about staying focused on "the work" in order to create a successful practice, I am challenging you to stay open to new ideas and new ways of working in order to expand your breadth of knowledge and scope of practice. This, more than anything, makes you more marketable.

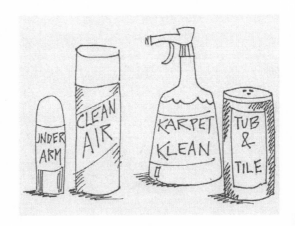

Golden Rule 4

Hygiene, Hygiene, Hygiene!

Image is important.
Think hair, nails, body odor, clothes, shoes, sheets, floor, carpet,
clutter, wastepaper basket, bathroom, bathroom, bathroom.

5. Getting Started

You've finished your formal education and are ready for clients. How you practice massage will be determined mostly by how you envision it, given your resources and resourcefulness.

> I would say, dream your dream, or other people will dream your dream for you. And to do that, you need to know who you are. Figure out who you are, figure out what you believe; don't take anyone's word for anything. Be skeptical. What the mind can conceive and the heart can believe, the body can achieve.
>
> Barry, Los Angeles, CA

With massage and alternative medical practices gaining more recognition and popularity, finding clients in even the most remote communities is becoming easier and easier. The public's perception of massage as a luxury service is fast being supplanted by their experience of massage as an integral part of general health and healing. Doctors of every persuasion are prescribing massage as an adjunct to their therapies. With the increased acceptance of massage in the medical community (not to mention the insurance business), it's not hard to convince the public of its benefits. Massage can also be pleasurable and a good way to simply relax, even in the absence of any specific health-related goals.

There are many decisions that need to be made before accepting clients. The first decision must be what type of massage you want to practice (see Appendix II, Massage Modalities). This will determine what kind of space and materials you will need. As you continue to grow your practice, your expertise will also grow, and decisions regarding your business will continue to change as well.

Full-Time or Part-Time?

Whether you have decided to practice massage full-time or part-time, in most cases, the beginning therapist needs to start slowly in order to build the strength and stamina required to do the work without injury. In some ways, it is more difficult for the part-time practitioner. Like the weekend warrior who is prone to injury (the athlete analogy again), the part-time therapist needs to work regularly to develop the strength and stamina required, precisely because it is a part-time endeavor. Pain is a good teacher. If doing massage causes pain, then reevaluation of body mechanics and table height are a good first response, followed by a dedicated regimen of strengthening and stretching exercises.

There is absolutely nothing wrong with wanting a part-time massage practice. A part-time practice may be the stepping stone to a full-time practice—just don't forget to allow time for building your strength and stamina. Good massage on any level should engage fully the body, the mind, and the spirit. Without the proper nourishment of each, a massage practice can be debilitating.

Where to work?

For many of us, one of the more attractive aspects of being a massage therapist is the ability to work on our own. Having this freedom and independence can be very rewarding, but generating and maintaining a business—marketing, returning phone calls, making appointments, ordering supplies, maintaining the space, keeping client and financial records—takes time and energy.

The other option, working for someone else, allows the therapist to focus full attention on the massage work and let someone else worry about the business end. Of course, there is a price to pay for this service—the proprietor takes a percentage of every fee. The employee therapist hopes to make up this lost income in tips, but of course there are no guarantees.

It is difficult to compare the advantages and disadvantages of working for someone else, because it involves so many diverse factors: whether you like the camaraderie of a larger workplace, your organizational and marketing skills, your need for downtime, and so on. Even comparing the profitability of being an employee therapist versus a self-employed one is difficult, requiring an evaluation of overhead expenses, tax deductions, and work flow.

> If you go work for somebody else, what is the value of the time, vacation pay, and insurance versus being on your own and paying the AMTA for insurance?
>
> Diane, New York, NY

Since I started practicing in 1992, the availability of massage has grown tremendously. Back then, one might find a massage therapist only at the higher-end gyms; now, it seems, people expect all gyms to provide this service. More and more people go to spas or spa hotels precisely because massage is available. Many chiropractors offer massage on their premises or refer their patients to a nearby therapist. Medical doctors and physical therapists, too, have begun to refer their patients to massage therapists. All of these environments offer the beginning therapist the opportunity to get bodies under their hands. Even if you aspire to working alone, a job with an established client base can afford valuable exposure to a number of clients with a range of conditions. Working part-time with a doctor, physical therapist, or a spa can help you build confidence, skill, strength, and stamina.

> Do two or three different jobs. Do part-time everywhere. Go work a couple of days a week at a spa, work for a chiropractic office, keep your own clientele, keep two or three personal clients a week, go somewhere for two days, go somewhere else for two days. You might like it. It might be chaotic. You might not want to work for yourself. At least the first year, do a few things. I'm not talking about job-hopping. I'm talking about making a commitment to be part-time at two or three different places.
>
> Diane, New York, NY

> The best thing you can do right out of school is go work someplace where you can get a lot of experience doing massage. There is so much to learn about the work: learning how to give a full session in a set amount of time, learning how much work your body can take, learning how to deal with the public, getting your body mechanics really working, building a reputation. It's a huge amount to assimilate all at once. The trick is finding a good environment, person, or business to work for.
>
> Theresa, Seattle, WA

Most spas or gyms are very specific about therapists not soliciting their clients for private sessions, which is understandable from a business point of view. Regulating where clients go for massage may seem silly. Massage is more than a service; it's about a relationship. People come for massage for lots of reasons, not the least of which is wanting to feel comfortable with the person to whom they are going to expose themselves. But the spa owner is also trying to develop a relationship with his or her customers and tries to provide them with convenience and familiarity. For therapists who aspire to having a private practice, honoring any contractual agreement with a spa owner is not only ethical but also sends a message to any potential private clients that we are professional and honorable.

Now, here is the sticking point for the spa owners. When a therapist leaves their employ, they hope the relationship they have forged with the customer is stronger than the one the therapist has cultivated. Regardless, the therapist is expected to walk away, breaking all contact with the customer. This is the part that seems unrealistic to me. It's the customer's decision to receive the work from whomever they choose. If the convenience of the spa supersedes the importance of the relationship with the therapist, the spa retains the customer. If not, the therapist has a private client. That is why employers often include noncompete and nonsolicitation clauses in their employees' contracts.

Noncompetition and Nonsolicitation Agreements
A noncompetition agreement can involve three different aspects: customers, geography, and information. The employer may hire the

employee therapist only if the employee agrees not to compete for customers, not to work elsewhere in the same vicinity (generally a five-mile radius) and/or not to disclose business, product, or client information. This is usually not a problem for the beginning therapist, but it may become a problem after you have established a reputation and a loyal following and consider leaving to start a private practice.

A nonsolicitation agreement stipulates that an employee therapist will not solicit business from the employer's customers privately, siphoning business from the employer. In effect, such an agreement also means that, even if a client solicits you to provide massage therapy privately, you must decline. If you have signed a nonsolicitation contract, a breach of the contract is a firing offense. But even in the absence of a contractual agreement, it is a breach of trust and usually ends in a parting of the ways. It is important for a therapist to always choose the ethical, professional path, especially if a noncompete or nonsolicitation contract was agreed to.

The same ethical approach should prevail for a noncompete clause. This type of agreement in an employer's contract prevents the therapist from competing for the same clients for a specific time period after leaving their employ. Building a practice requires forging relationships based on trust and honesty. Even if a client chooses to stay with the spa for reasons of convenience, they will always remember your work and professional behavior and may recommend you to their friends.

Spa Work

The spa industry is the largest employer of massage therapists in the country. Day spas seem to have sprouted in every community, forcing the beauty industry to rethink the quality and menu of services they offer their customers. The massage therapist is the happy beneficiary of this growth but also in many cases the slave to its corporate management and mismanagement. Massage therapists are full of stories of working long, underappreciated, and underpaid hours in spas where the primary goal is to herd clients like cattle in and out of massage rooms. Having had a massage studio that supports several massage therapists in Manhattan, I am well aware of the huge expense involved in running a massage establishment, and so I don't want to feed the impression that the little guy is always taken advantage of by the money-hungry business owner. Some of the more enlightened spa owners realize that happy and healthy employees translate into better customer satisfaction and less time and money spent on recruitment and training. Yet far too often, spas are run by corporate managers who focus only on the bottom line. Most of these managers have little or no actual massage experience with which to relate to the workhorse of the operation, the therapist. The health of the therapists, if on their radar screen at all, is near the bottom of the owner's priorities. (Realistically, though, if a company isn't structured to make money, then it will not survive, and neither will the jobs it provides. This is not an original problem, and it is played out in the business world every day.) Though many spas espouse the importance of working as a team, seldom have I heard a therapist speak positively about this work ethic. More often, it is a lack of teamwork that sends a therapist packing. With the spa industry still in its infancy and lacking a unifying labor union, the therapist's only power is in choosing not to work for disreputable business owners.

Despite all this, working in this kind of establishment has its advantages, especially for the beginning therapist. First and foremost, the spa provides a steady flow of customers and a place to gain experience, to build strength and stamina, and to network and forge new business relationships. The spa becomes the apprentice workshop or internship for the neophyte therapist. The spa industry has brought massage therapy to the masses and given the profession a much higher profile, and for that we should all be grateful. But we need to be participants in the growth of our industry so we are not simply cogs in a machine but a vital part of the success of the business. Doing good work gives us that power. The satisfied customer translates into more business for the business owner and, one hopes, an appreciative employer (if not, then consider moving on).

It's important to enter the spa world with realistic expectations and, more importantly, realistic goals. For the therapist who doesn't like to compromise and prefers working alone, spa work is probably an exercise in anxiety-provoking futility. Bear in mind, too, that your goals may change over time and you may need to reevaluate and redefine them.

Give yourself permission to change your mind, your goals, and your job. Think of each job as a learning experience, an opportunity to refine your massage skills, your people skills, and your business skills.

Striking Out on Your Own

Whether you have just left school or spent years working for others, committing to a private practice can be frightening. For someone who has never worked alone, losing the security and benefits of working for someone else can feel like jumping off a cliff. In order to fly, though, you must first jump. Over the years I have heard countless stories of massage therapists (myself included) looking at their empty appointment books in distress. The only solution to this is to reaffirm your faith in your work and in the universe to provide for you, followed by a consistent plan of action. Once you implement this, you will find that somehow, at the end of the week, you actually met new clients and made money. In other words, relax, take a deep breath, and stick to the plan. Take the next step.

> I'm happily self-employed, but it's not for everyone. You have to be comfortable with a malleable structure to your days. I think if you want to be a successful therapist working for others, you have to really be willing to put in the work, protect your boundaries and ethics, be clear about what you are willing and not willing to do, and keep your expectations reasonable.
>
> Theresa, Seattle, WA

The next step is deciding where to work. You will need to consider who your market or target audience is, but first, let's explore all the options.

Deciding Where to Work

Choices that don't involve renting or buying space include:

Working in hotels or spas
Making house calls
On-site business
Working from home

Options that involve renting or buying a space include:

Establishing your own space
Establishing a space with other therapists or health-care professionals
Renting space from a doctor, physical therapist, or other health professional

House Calls

House calls present their own set of considerations. In general, the overhead expenses are lower, but you must also consider the added time and expense of traveling. This time and expense is generally passed on to the client in the way of a higher fee for house calls. Clients expect to pay a higher fee for the convenience, but there is a limit to what they will spend for travel time. Some therapists tack on a variable travel expense to their regular fee, while others have a flat rate for all house calls that covers average travel time.

Safety can also be a concern with house calls. For a first-time client, it's a good idea to let someone know where you are going and when you will be finished. This communication can even be conducted in front of the client before starting. This is when a cell phone is an extremely useful tool. When entering a client's residence, always pay attention to where the exits are and always trust your instincts. If a situation feels uncomfortable or even slightly dangerous, do your best to apologize and excuse yourself. Keeping a cell phone handy for an emergency call is a good idea.

> The biggest pitfall for therapists is not listening to their instincts. The only times I've had difficulties is when I override my instincts about that. You can tell on the phone what people are interested in. Make sure you are safe. I've often thought about working at home, but I've decided I'm much more comfortable keeping my home and my business separate. It doesn't have as much to do with safety as it does with keeping things clear. I'm very clear about what is going on in my work space.
>
> Peggy, Melbourne, FL

Hotel Work

Most hotel work involves a relationship with the concierge, who essentially wants a cut of the fee for referring his hotel guests to us. In general, we're talking about higher-end hotels, so the fee is generally higher than even the standard house call. The concierge wants two things: to keep his guests happy and to maximize his tips, whether these come from the guest or the therapist. Customer satisfaction and even loyalty might play into the equation, but unless the client specifically asks for you, a concierge is likely to call the therapist who pays him the largest fee and who is available when the client requests. Being "on call" for hotel work can complicate scheduling the rest of your life.

Hotel work might be a good choice for a therapist who likes to work irregular hours and late nights, or perhaps one who lives in a tourist area. But hotel work is highly dependent on tourism and the business traveler, so if the economy takes a turn for the worse, the therapist who depends largely on the hotel client for income will suffer more than one with a more diverse client base. The primary benefit to hotel work is a higher income, since hotel guests are accustomed to paying a premium for this "luxury." Since the concierge is the gatekeeper to your success, you pay to cultivate this relationship. It is hard to know what the appropriate or smart tip is in order to get his attention. This type of tipping is highly subjective. It is probably just as important to make his job easy for him by providing contact information, the days and hours you are available, and business cards. This is where a professional-looking flyer with all the pertinent information can come in handy. In essence, the concierge is your employer, and a friendly, professional, and amiable demeanor is imperative for getting his attention and his phone call. Being on call in this way requires consistent, dependable access and an almost immediate response time in order to grow this relationship and this part of your business.

On-Site Business

Another share of the massage business that is highly dependent on the health of the economy is on-site therapy. This is essentially chair massage done in the business community, though not exclusively. My company ran a modestly successful on-site business during the dot-com boom of the 1990s—until the crash, when all the corporate money for such things disappeared. Nonetheless, therapists are finding the chair massage business to be a burgeoning part of the industry and are setting up chairs anywhere from street fairs and airports to convention centers and boardrooms. In addition, therapists are using the public visibility of chair massage to establish relationships with the community and foster new clients.

Establishing Your Own Business

Finding and creating a commercial space that is suitable and comfortable for practicing massage may take a little time and money and a lot of imagination. Venturing into this part of the business requires some foresight, a business plan, creativity, and even some luck. Starting any new business is a gamble, betting that our investment of time, money, talent, and resources will net a profit. The best insurance against the unknown is careful planning. It might be a good idea to work for other massage establishments first in order to observe the day-to-day operation of the business.

Observing and experiencing what the customer experiences in order to fully evaluate the service being provided is also a good idea. The best way to get valuable information, whether from the customer's or the business owner's perspective, is to observe and listen. Asking questions at the appropriate time can also be helpful, though some business owners, fearing competition, may be reluctant to divulge too much information regarding their operation.

Not all talented massage therapists are also talented business people. If you are not, get some help in drawing up your business plan—perhaps from a lawyer or an accountant, or from a massage therapist who has already established a business. Arriving at your own business plan will take some thought. Here are some basic questions to help you get started.

Checklist: Making a Business Plan

1. Will your business be a sole proprietorship or a corporation?

Incorporating has some legal and financial benefits that may make the expense worth the investment, but it also entails certain tax-reporting requirements that may be time consuming. An accountant and lawyer will best be able to advise you on this question.

2. Will you work alone or will you have employees?

3. Will the people who work with you be employees or independent contractors?

The IRS defines an independent contractor by the amount of control the employer exerts over the person doing the work. The general rule of thumb is that an independent contractor's work (the result) can be determined by the employer, but not the means or methods for accomplishing the result. If you hire an independent contractor and pay him or her more than $600 in a calendar year, you must report this to the IRS at the end of the year. An employee, on the other hand, is someone whose work can be controlled by the employer, as well as how the work is to be accomplished. If you have employees, you must withhold city, state, and federal income taxes, file quarterly tax reports, and pay social security, Medicare, and unemployment taxes. An accountant can help you navigate through the various forms required.

4. Will you need a receptionist or bookkeeper?

5. What are the start-up expenses and ongoing expenses for the new company?

6. What is a comfortable and affordable rent?

7. Is there a lease?

8. Are utilities included in the rent?

9. Will you have twenty-four-hour access to the space?

10. How much space do you need, including storage?

11. Is there a private bathroom in the space or a shared one?

12. Does the bathroom have a shower, and do you want to offer that convenience?

13. Do you want walk-in traffic, and does your office support that?

14. Will the neighborhood feel safe for clients both during the day and at night?

15. Is safe parking available for people who drive?

16. What is the basic list and cost of supplies and materials you need to get started?

17. What is the basic list and cost of furniture and office equipment you need to get started?

18. How much insurance beyond basic liability insurance do you need?

19. How and where will you advertise?

20. How much financial reserve will you need to get through the start-up process or through a slow period?

21. How will you bring in clients, and what is your marketing plan? What is your backup plan?

Navigating through all the business aspects can be a daunting experience, but it is important to consider them all. Just as important are service-oriented questions that will define the product and how it is delivered, like the following.

Checklist: Defining Your Product

1. What services will you offer? Products?

2. What materials and equipment do you need to provide these services?

3. What kind of atmosphere do you want to create?

You might spend some time visiting different spas and massage establishments to see what already exists in your community. Observe your competition and try to clearly define your strengths and that which will make your establishment unique while also trying to minimize your weaknesses. Even though businesses compete for clients, there is room for all of us to be successful. As health-care practitioners, we need to perceive and support other massage businesses as colleagues and comrades rather than solely as competition. We are all part of a community network of bodywork professionals. It is this network of like-minded professionals that will serve to advertise our presence in the community.

Sharing a Space

Setting up a space with another health-care professional like a chiropractor or acupuncturist has its advantages and disadvantages. The most obvious advantage is that expenses, and often clients, can be shared. The greatest disadvantage is loss of autonomy. Business associates, like family members, require a certain degree of understanding and compromise in order for the relationship to work. (Friends and family members, by the way, don't necessarily make the best business associates, because each role has different boundaries for appropriate behavior.) The most important consideration is to clearly define all aspects of the professional relationship *in writing,* and it's a good idea to have a lawyer review this document. If one partner has an existing practice, then some of the practical decisions in terms of use of space have already been determined. In this instance, the new partner may simply be a tenant who pays rent to the established partner. It is still important to clearly define the parameters for use of the space, including common areas, storage areas, restrooms, and hours of availability and operation. The terms of the lease, whether for a tenant or for a partner, should clearly outline how and when the rent is to be paid and whether it is a monthly lump sum or a percentage of each client; whether there is a security deposit, what it covers, how it is returned at the end of the lease, and what happens in case of default. You need to define in a written business agreement how utilities are paid; how equipment and supplies are obtained and maintained; what office equipment is required or available to each party and how it is maintained (including phone, fax, answering machine, copy machine, computer, printer, and files); what liability each party has for the lease and the physical space in terms of repair or personal injury; how much liability insurance is required for each party; how to handle disagreements; and, just as important, how to end the relationship equitably and amicably.

There are multitudes of ways to partner and share a space, each with benefits and downsides. A major benefit is sharing resources. A benefit for practitioners who are not practicing the same modality is increased access to potential clients. A downside for practitioners of the same modality is competition for the same clients or even a feeling of jealousy when one practitioner is busier. On the other hand, more established and secure practitioners might like being able to refer clients to their partner when they are sick or on vacation.

For the health of the relationship, it is vitally important to consider, negotiate, and outline in writing a signed agreement on how the partnership will operate and even how it will dissolve. Even with the best intentions, people can easily or conveniently forget or change their minds about a venture that initially seems viable but in practice becomes unworkable.

> It's very hard to go into business with someone with whom you are a close friend. There should be paperwork—my responsibilities, your responsibilities. We agreed to this, it's signed and dated. It's not to take anyone to court; it's so that in an objective way, if someone's not meeting their responsibilities, we can say, "You agreed to this." And it doesn't wind up being an emotional thing or a personal thing. It's just an agreement.
>
> Tamara, Chicago, IL

Working from Home

For some therapists, working from home is a perfect solution to bearing the strain of establishing a private practice. It's obvious that choosing a practice that doesn't involve renting space lowers the operating cost of the business. Without this added expense, you will have more resources and time to devote to your budding practice. In addition, the expense of commuting to work is eliminated. Best of all, when you work from home, you are the master and commander of your own environment. You set the schedule, run your ship as you see fit, and split your fee with no one.

There are, however, some important things to consider before setting up a practice in the living room or spare bedroom. First, you need to check zoning laws and procure any license that may be required. Your city or county's zoning commission is a good first step for identifying zoning limitations. Try searching online by entering your city and state followed by the suffix ".gov" and then searching "home business," "zoning," and "licensing" links. The Small Business Administration at www.sba.gov is a good resource, as are www.business.gov and www. smallbusiness.gov. Other community and zoning concerns you may need to consider are hours of operation, signage, and rental property usage versus home ownership usage. Some residential areas restrict the operation of small businesses in order to limit the increased parking, traffic, and noise. Of course, requesting a zoning variance is an option, but it may require an application fee and navigating through city or county agencies for the proper protocol.

Next, it's a good idea to consult with a lawyer or accountant to determine what type of business entity is best for you: a sole-proprietorship, a corporation, or perhaps even a partnership if you are starting a business with someone. A business lawyer or accountant can define the benefits of incorporating and even which type of corporation to form. Each has different benefits and liabilities and will require some deliberation.

Many state, county, and local governments require companies to obtain a business license. Requirements vary by locale. A local lawyer can help with this process; there are also businesses that help new companies expedite this process. A simple web search for "business license" will provide multiple licensing service companies that can help you navigate this process. If you plan to sell merchandise, you will need to obtain a reseller's certificate. Another web search will help you with this process.

Working from home does not preclude the need for liability insurance. Along with professional liability insurance, which most practitioners obtain by joining a professional organization like the AMTA (American Massage Therapy Association), casualty and property insurance are a good idea. Casualty insurance supplements property insurance, though they are often referred to together as "property and casualty" insurance. Essentially, property insurance insures the location, while casualty insurance insures the business. If you are working from home, consulting an insurance broker will help you define what will be covered by your home owner's policy and what additional coverage you may need to cover your business. There are multitudes of insurance products, like disability insurance, business continuation, and business interruption insurance. You may want to explore with an insurance broker to determine what is best for you.

For some, working from home may not allow a large enough separation between business and personal life. But if you do work from home, having a separate workspace within your home helps establish boundaries for both you and your clients. A separate, dedicated workspace also makes it easier to take a tax deduction for a percentage of your rent or mortgage payments and utilities.

For female therapists, especially, safety should be a primary concern. That's not to say that male practitioners are not in danger of malfeasance. For some therapists, male or female, the threat of a sexual predator or simply an invasion of privacy may preclude working from home as a viable option. There are "tricks of the trade" that therapists use to help overcome the sexual threat. When receiving clients at home, you might leave a radio or television on in another room to give the impression that someone else is present. Talking to someone (who is not actually there) within earshot of the client sends the same message. Ending a telephone conversation with someone explaining that your new client is arriving can also be effective.

Despite its disadvantages, receiving clients at home can add a personal touch to the work. You just need to make sure that it is a clean and professional touch as well. Not everyone has the same idea of what clean and sanitary means, especially when we consider the bathroom. Let's just say that nothing is too clean. Consider, too, the smells in your home. While cooking smells like fish, garlic, or even fresh-baked bread may be delicious to some, they may seem off-putting or inappropriate to others.

In general, pets preclude working from home. I am speaking of the furry, four-legged, allergy-inducing variety. What some consider the most precious creatures on earth others may see as a sneezing, dripping, allergenic nightmare. And litter boxes or birdcages are not anyone's idea of aromatherapy. Talking birds, not to mention a wayward reptile or rodent, can prove to be a client-losing proposition.

The work space, whether it is an integral part of your living space or not, should have a very distinct and professional feel to it. It should be clear to clients what space is available to them, allowing especially for privacy while undressing. Speaking of privacy, keep in mind that clients may go exploring (the contents of your closet or your medicine cabinet, for instance). You may want to consider relocating personal effects to a place that is off limits to your clients.

Finally, consider what additional furniture or equipment you will need for your home office. In addition to the requisite massage table and linens, you need to consider how and where you will store client files and business receipts. You may want a separate office computer, printer, phone, and answering machine. You will need shelving for storage of linens, cream, oil, and equipment in addition to lighting and music. You will also need to consider furniture for your clients to use while undressing and for hanging their clothes or placing their belongings while they are receiving massage and perhaps even a mirror for them to use while dressing afterward. An area rug is a nice touch, especially in the winter.

Checklist: Setting Up a Home-Based Business

1. Check zoning laws regarding home businesses

Go to your local city or county zoning commission or "your city".gov.

2. Establish your business entity

Consult your lawyer or accountant about setting up a sole proprietorship, partnership, or corporation.

3. Obtain business licenses

Check state requirements; also obtain reseller's certificate if selling merchandise.

4. Obtain proper insurance

Determine how much insurance you need beyond basic liability insurance. Do you need or want professional and personal liability insurance? Property and casualty insurance? Business continuation or interruption insurance? Disability insurance?

5. Define dedicated office space and hours

Determine the percentage of your home being used for professional purposes, for tax deductions.

6. Define equipment needed

    a. Work equipment: table, stool, and supplies
    b. Office equipment: phone, computer, shelves, etc.
    c. Client furniture: chair, table, mirror, etc.

Buying a Table

The most common modality in which a massage table is required is Swedish massage. Choosing the right table for massage is as important as it is for a pianist to choose the right piano. Even this seemingly simple decision requires some deliberation. Will the table be stationary or will it be used to make house calls? If so, you will want to consider its weight and portability.

Generally, the heavier the table, the greater working weight it can bear. (Working weight is the weight of the client plus the force and weight applied by the practitioner. Static weight indicates the weight of the client lying still on the table.) The width of the table is also a consideration. A standard width is twenty-nine to thirty inches, but tables can range from twenty-five to thirty-three inches. Shorter practitioners may have more difficulty reaching across a wider table. Wider clients will feel uncomfortable on smaller tables. A greater width also adds more weight.

The standard height of a massage table is twenty-four to thirty-four inches. Taller practitioners will generally want a taller table. The standard rule of thumb here is that the table should reach your knuckles when you are standing with arms extended at the side of the table, but I often advise students to adjust the table down to fingertip height. This allows you to work in a squatted position, effectively lowering your center of gravity and facilitating leaning rather than pressing (see chapter 10, Self-Care). The average padding adds another 2-1/2 to 3 inches. More padding adds more comfort for the client but also adds more weight and more expense.

Aluminum tables tend to be lighter than wood and are more expensive, though my experience with metal tables is that they squeak over time. A wood table can also squeak, but tightening the screws and in some cases applying a bit of oil or wax can easily solve the problem. Some aluminum tables have telescoping legs that make adjusting height easier but can be more expensive, while some tables have fully collapsible legs so the table can sit directly on the floor. This feature allows the therapist to work on the floor, as with shiatsu or Thai massage. Realistically, though, working in this way can be very awkward and uncomfortable for the practitioner—it is easier to simply use a thick carpet or pad for floor massage techniques.

Auto-lock support systems are generally more expensive because of the ease of their setup compared to tables that require a two- to four-step leg-locking assembly. End access panels and side cables that give the legs support are also worth considering. Most table manufacturers realize that the therapist sits at the ends and sides of the table to work, and so end plates and cables are usually constructed to allow space for the therapist's knees. Cheaper models, however, sometimes lack this space.

Some cheaper tables only have holes to attach the face cradle at one end and so are less versatile. Face cradles themselves come in many different versions. As with any machine, the more moving parts there are, the more likely the product will need maintenance and repair. The more adjustable the face cradle is, though, the more it can be suited to different clients' needs, particularly clients with limited neck flexibility or large-breasted women.

The table cover and color are also worth considering. Even though the table is always draped with linen, choosing its cover color can elicit hours of deliberation. Often less popular colors that a company may have in stock are offered at a discount. Cover materials are generally synthetics like nylon or polyurethane, but more eco-friendly materials (as well as tables made of wood with water-based lacquers and glues) are now becoming available. One might also consider the nap of the material. Unfitted sheets can easily move when clients turn over on smoother covers, while a material that has a degree of nap holds the sheet in place. Reinforced corners can also add to the price of the table but add durability to the cover. A table cover or carrying case is a very good idea, even if traveling is not part of your business plan. Protecting the table against unwanted wear and tear while storing affords it the respect it deserves. A therapist with his table in the shop is like a pianist without her piano. The music stops, and so does the paycheck.

There are numerous accessories that can add to the versatility and comfort of a table. Tilt-top tables and hydraulic lifts make tables more accommodating for older and infirm clients, but they require more room, are difficult to move, and are much more expensive. Some tables come with removable breast and pregnancy inserts. These options can be useful for some clients, but they add expense, and the breast options don't accommodate all women. Fleece covers for the table and face cradle add padding, warmth, and comfort. Egg-crate foam can be placed on top of a table, allowing for less built-in foam and reducing the cost and the weight of the table. Table warmers or electric blankets, especially in the winter, add comfort and relaxation. Arm extensions can be added to accommodate wider clients.

Money, of course, is a major determining factor when buying a table. Lighter tables (aluminum or soft top) tend to be more expensive and often have a more limited warranty. Heavier tables are more likely to have a longer warranty. Let me suggest the possibility that you may want a new table after a few years. New designs are introduced every year, so a lifetime warranty may not be worth the extra expense. You may also grow to hate teal or burgundy. Buying a used table to start is a good idea. It introduces you to a brand of table, gets you working on a table less expensively, and allows you to determine what features are more important to you before investing a larger sum of money.

Checklist: Choosing a Table

1. Stationary vs. traveling

2. Height and width

3. Foam layer

4. Weight
    a. working surface dimensions
    b. aluminum vs. wood legs
    c. wood vs. soft top
    d. portability
    e. foam thickness

5. Ease of assembly
    a. auto-lock legs
    b. telescoping legs
    c. collapsible legs (for shiatsu or floor work)

6. Double-end face cradle option

7. Cover
    a. nap
    b. reinforced corners
    c. color

8. Options
    a. tilt-top or hydraulic lift
    b. pregnancy/breast inserts
    c. fleece cover
    d. egg-crate foam
    e. table warmer
    f. arm rests/arm extensions
    g. carrying case

9. Price

10. Warranty

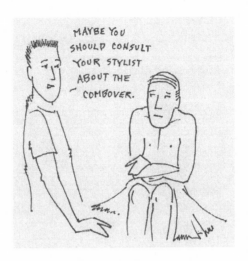

Golden Rule 5

Practice what you preach.

Speaking from a place of experience confers credibility.
Be careful, though, of the advice you offer—your clients may listen.
Keep it within the scope of the profession.

6. Pricing

For some aspiring therapists, the prospect of making a lot of money brings them to the profession. The general thinking goes something like this: "If one massage nets $75 an hour, then a forty-hour week will net $3,000.00. There are four weeks in a month and twelve months in a year—ka-ching, ka-ching. Wow, there's money to be made in massage!" For any working therapist, this thought process is nothing but ludicrous. There are many attractive reasons to get involved in the field of massage, and money may be one of them. But I think I can safely say that getting rich and doing forty massages in a week is not at all near anyone's reality in the profession. The actual number of hands-on massage hours a therapist can do week after week depends on many factors, including age, physical fitness, type of work, and ongoing commitment to self-care—but a more realistic range is ten to twenty hours of massage per week. Bear in mind, too, that for every hour of massage, there can easily be two hours of marketing, record keeping, maintenance, and self-care in order to sustain a healthy client-centered practice.

> I got paid twenty-five dollars for house calls. I thought I was making a fortune. Unfortunately, you don't work forty hours a week, and you quickly learn you're not making a fortune; you're just making a lot per hour.
>
> Alexis, Wainscott, NY

Determining Price

At the start of every therapist's career comes the task of putting a monetary value to the work. It is not long before the ego gets entangled in this thought process and even the most self-assured individual confronts the question "What am I worth?" It is important not to confuse the monetary value of your work with self-value. It is natural for any therapist (and not necessarily just the beginning therapist) to invest in wanting clients to like their work. A logical association to follow is wanting the client to like the therapist himself. (Remember Sally Field's Academy Award acceptance speech: "You *like* me, you really *like* me!"?) This is a place where each therapist needs to explore the concept of boundaries. Certainly you want your clients to like you. I guarantee that if a client doesn't like you, the relationship will not be long-lived. Here again, the focus needs to be on the work. If your intention is to do good work, it will help to protect your ego from the whims of your clients. Establishing a price can be an emotional endeavor, and the clearer you are with your motivations, your intentions, and your boundaries, the less emotionally charged the decision will be.

> If you give yourself permission to ask a certain fee for what you do, you're telling that person, "I value myself to the degree that I know that I'm worth this."
>
> Barry, Los Angeles, CA

From a marketing perspective, generally we think the best or lowest price wins. This standard may be sound for air conditioners and automobiles, but not in the service industry. In the service industry, how a product or service is delivered can be as important as the product itself.

We're also familiar with the concept that "you get what you pay for." Ultimately, though, I think the quality of the work determines the price. It is difficult to determine the value one receives from massage. Two therapists of equal skill and style may have a completely different value to a client based on their conversational skills or social interests. To a particular client, having company and conversation may be of more value than a good massage. So the massage therapist who views socializing during a massage as a boundary not to cross would probably have less value to that particular client. The client who wants to communicate as little as possible and simply "get to the rub" might place a greater value on the other therapist. The good therapist is flexible to the client's needs (client-centered) and determines those by listening to the client's text and subtext and getting the client to communicate their needs. This leads to a strengthened relationship. It's the relationship that enhances the value of our work. Of course, there are many criteria for determining value and price, and we could fill a room with successful therapists and debate for hours. Instead, I'll list a few pointers that might facilitate your process.

1. Determine the price range for massage in your area.
Simply visit the local yellow pages or Internet listings and inquire about services and prices. The American Massage Therapy Association has a website (www.amtamassage.com) where one can find a therapist by locale.

2. Sample different massages in your area.
Check out the competition. It is probably a good idea to get massages in a variety of settings both public and private to determine what therapists and massage establishments are charging for their services. It's also a way to learn about all aspects of your work, from pricing to technique. It's not a bad idea for the beginning therapist to sample other modalities, not only in the realm of massage but also in alternate modalities like chiropractic or physical therapy as well. This research (which is tax-deductible) will provide not only an experiential knowledge of other modalities but also a network of colleagues for referral. Do not underestimate the value of this network. Networking begins with a network.

Your research can serve another purpose, as well. While receiving the work, consider the practitioner's skill, comfort, atmosphere, responsiveness, location, personality, professionalism, and finally, the fee. All of these aspects help to determine or support your price.

> What I try to do now is ask a lot of other therapists in the area what they charge, and then I practice saying things like, "My fee is ninety dollars an hour." I have to practice it, say it out loud. I don't know what I am worth in money terms. That's an issue that's very difficult for me to deal with. Money has always been a struggle for me.
>
> Alexis, Wainscott, NY

3. Ask colleagues and friends for feedback.
Ask colleagues what they are charging for massage and how they decided
on their fee. Most therapists love to talk about their work and are eager
to share their wisdom. You might even ask your friends what they pay
for massage or, more importantly, what they are willing to pay. This
information can be valuable when determining price. Finally, though,
any feedback, especially from nonprofessionals, needs to be considered
in the larger context of your own particular needs and goals.

Sliding Scales

For the beginning therapist trying to build a practice, losing a client
because the fee is too high can be disheartening. Offering a sliding scale,
for some, is the answer. At first glance, this seems an ideal solution:
the client gets the work at an affordable price, and the therapist's ego
and bank account are enriched. I mention ego again because inevitably
when we compromise our fee, at some point in our relationship with this
client, we will have to confront our self-worth demon again. Initially
the ego is stroked because we have another client to call our own.
It's when we have many clients or perhaps when this client becomes
"difficult" that the dark side of the ego begins talking to us. Let me
start by saying emphatically that no matter what the compromise is,
you need to be able to walk away and feel satisfied with your decision.
It is not fair to punish the client for either their economic status or
for your poor negotiating skills. Though the fee may be reduced, the
work should never be compromised. If at any point you feel taken
advantage of because of a compromised fee, you need to take a minute
to reevaluate the benefit of having this client. If you find it difficult to
justify a negotiated fee, renegotiate.

What we cannot afford to do is resent a client for paying us less than we
think we are worth. This resentment, no matter how cleverly disguised,
will at some point manifest in our work and our relationship with
the client. For example, we may feel justified in giving a fifty-five-
minute massage instead of the contracted sixty. Remember that we
are developing relationships. Relationships require communication.
Communicating with compassion can help you navigate through a
potentially difficult and perhaps embarrassing negotiation. Discussing
money can be difficult for both the therapist and the client. (The

difficulty of handling such situations is one reason some therapists choose not to start a private practice. Instead, working for someone else allows you to focus on the work while the management handles the business end.) Finding a network of colleagues or a mentor with whom you can discuss and work through some of the difficulties of skillful communication can be an invaluable asset in trying to successfully manage a practice.

> I offered a sliding scale in the beginning, as I was building my confidence. It was a way to build in a learning curve, like being able to take a little pressure off. I feel that the new students, the beginners, can offer a low rate. It's really important to line up what you are asking with your skill level and what you feel is appropriate.
>
> Denise, San Francisco, CA

Other things to consider regarding a sliding scale include determining who is eligible for the reduced rate, when they stop being eligible, or how to handle a reduced-rate increase. Everyone enjoys a bargain. Explaining to clients why they are or are not eligible for a rate reduction can be uncomfortable for everyone. This can be especially difficult if a client with a reduced rate refers a friend to you. It is a good policy, therefore, to request that clients who receive a reduced rate not advertise this to their friends. You might suggest that you are happy that you are able to offer them a reduced rate but that it is your regular rate that allows you to offer a few clients this benefit.

> There have been times when I have resented a client because I charged them less. But I should be annoyed with myself, not with them. They're paying me what I asked for.
>
> Alexis, Wainscott, NY

Certainly it is easier to have one fee for all clients. It helps avoid having to deal with a lot of difficult situations. Balancing the desire to help people with our need to make our business profitable is a constant battle for all health-care professionals. Remember, though, that having enough money to live on is a huge part of taking care of ourselves. Our clients look to us as role models. If we are always exhausted because we are working too much, not only will our work suffer, but we also lose some of our credibility as professionals.

Before considering a sliding scale, spend some time evaluating your financial needs. This is the benefit of a business plan, even when you are running your own business. It gives you some perspective and gets you out of the emotional realm when making important financial decisions. If you look at money and payment for services as a boundary issue (see chapter 9, Boundaries), it's easier to understand the complexity of pricing. Boundaries, even without the added emotional weight of money, require clear communication and articulation, first for us and then for our clients.

Raising Your Fee

It may seem like an odd time to think about a fee increase when you are just establishing a practice, but it's worth considering. At some point in your career, you will want to raise your fee, and it may be better to set the fee slightly higher now to reduce the frequency of increases. For some therapists, balancing the need for a raise with the impression of not being greedy can be difficult. If you start your practice with a low fee with the idea of raising it in the near future, you will confront this issue sooner rather than later—and it can be difficult to raise fees, especially for clients on fixed incomes. Certainly, if your fee is lower, your services will be more available to more people. When it is time to raise your fee, though, you will have to confront the very people for whom you made the accommodation.

Balancing the choice of providing your services for those who need them and those who can afford them is never easy. This might be a time to consider the sliding-scale approach. Suggesting another therapist who charges less is also an option.

One way to help your clients absorb the news of a rate increase is a well-written letter describing the need for one. Most clients understand that over time, we need to raise our rates to adjust for the cost of living.

Sending a letter a few months before the increase allows your clients to not only adjust their budgets but also to adjust psychologically. Include in your letter the date of your last rate increase, the amount of the increase, and the date for the pending increase. (I often include wit or humor in the letter, or maybe a famous quote, to soften the news.) You might also consider what time of year is best for clients to accommodate to the increase, both financially and psychologically. Though the beginning of a new year seems a natural beginning point for a rate increase, many people are also trying to absorb the expense of the holidays at that point. On the other hand, this may be when some of your clients receive bonuses at work. What's best for your clients will depend on their individual situations.

Try a psychological approach. This is an absolutely elitist approach but certainly worth considering, especially if you are working with elite or wealthy clients (when in Rome …). There is a psychological perception that if the fee for a service is high, then the service is good. By extension, if the service is limited (because the therapist is busy or popular) then the service must be good. This is a bit of a gamble, especially when you are sitting at home waiting for the phone to ring. And it is only an effective strategy if the work is in fact good. This brings us back to the recurring theme: *focus on the work!*

Pricing your services can be fraught with emotional, self-worth, self-care, and boundary issues. Taking the time to examine all of these issues both within your practice and within your personal life can only facilitate the ease with which you comport yourself in both arenas. For some therapists, this may not be a major issue. For others, I suggest practicing the vocabulary of pricing on friends and colleagues to begin getting comfortable with the idea of asking people for recompense. We absolutely have to separate our person from our work, but it is impossible to place value on our work if we do not first value ourselves.

Bartering

Exchanging services is a common form of recompense in the world of massage. Besides the pitfalls of circumventing the IRS (check the IRS website, www.irs.gov, for details), there are a few things to be aware of before venturing into this seemingly fortuitous arrangement. When cash flow is low and another service provider is willing, bartering services seems a good idea. But as with any financial arrangement, defining and clearly articulating terms is imperative in order to keep the relationship healthy. Ideally, each party should assign a clear value to the service being provided and then negotiate the terms. Keep in mind that value is subjective. Not all products are equal in their dollar-for-dollar value. For some people, the service that is exchanged may have a higher perceived value because of some other factor like convenience or need.

Besides the monetary value, the time and place of the services provided should be considered. Is there a time limit or expiration date on the services? Is travel time involved? If you are offering a series of massages, is there a date by which the services must be rendered or forfeited? Can the recipient give his massages to other people? If the services expand or change, how are the terms to be renegotiated? If the scope of the exchange involves multiple massages over a long period of time, a written contract is not a bad idea. Keeping an accurate account of rendered services is imperative.

Once you have agreed to the terms of a barter arrangement, it is important to follow through and honor them. More than anything, we need to give each massage the professional attention and dedication we would give to a paying client. Many therapists discover over time that paying for services rendered is the easiest, least complicated, and most efficient way of payment.

> I barter with the woman who works at the laundry a block away. But I do it very selectively. In the beginning I did a lot of barter work because I didn't have any money. But mostly, bartering is too complicated.
>
> Tamara, Chicago, IL

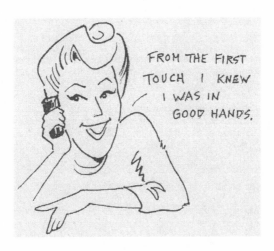

Golden Rule 6

Never forget the power of touch!

Imagine what your touch feels like throughout the massage.
Make it compassionate and effective.

7. Marketing

Any good book on starting a business has to have a chapter on marketing. And any chapter on marketing needs to talk about a business plan. For most people who have never been in business, the idea of creating a business plan can be daunting, if not downright scary. So first let me say that a business plan can be as simple or as complicated as you want or need it to be. For the most part, though, a business plan needs to account for your income and expenses so that you end up with a profit (for a checklist on making your business plan, see chapter 5).

Marketing, though, is much more than a good business plan. It is the process of taking a product to the marketplace for sale. There are several steps involved in going to market with a product:

Developing the product
Setting goals for selling the product
Packaging the product
Advertising

Developing the Product

Without a good product, no amount of marketing will be successful. Here again, "It's about the work." Our education is the developmental phase of our product preparation. Massage is no longer just a recreational luxury. In order to be competitive and successful, the increasingly informed public has come to expect massage therapists to help them both relax and rehabilitate. A comprehensive education with a strong foundation in anatomy, physiology, and pathology is required in order to speak the language of the body, in which the public itself is more and more conversant. We never stop our educational process. Our product is continually developing and changing. We need to constantly work on our technique and our artistry to keep the work vital, current, and interesting. If our work doesn't continue to grow, we grow bored with the work and our clients grow bored with our product. Conversely, there are those clients who don't like variety and who want to know what to expect. For them, we need to be sensitive to their expectations and introduce change in small increments. From a purely business perspective, this translates to giving the client what they want.

Successful businesses are constantly looking at ways to improve their products to better stay current and competitive in the ever-changing marketplace. Our product is our work, and it is nurtured by a curious mind and a conscientious approach to continuing education. There are different ways to pursue this continuing education: for some therapists, learning different modalities is a stimulating endeavor that keeps us fresh and, for the client, is like adding new products. Other therapists might prefer to focus on one modality and work to become an expert in that field. In either case, staying current and informed about what the marketplace offers keeps us competitive.

Setting Goals

Setting goals is about vision: making those decisions that inform the type of practice we want, setting goals to achieve them, outlining individual steps to reach each goal. With all goals, whether long- or short-term, it is important to outline the individual steps to achieve them. It helps to write them down, so that over time you can remind yourself of your goals, evaluate your progress, and make adjustments. This is the same process we follow when formulating a business plan, just broader in scope. For example:

Decision: I want to set up a part-time private practice in my home.

Goal: I want to average five clients per week within a year.

Steps: Convert the spare bedroom by the end of month
 First week
   Clear and paint room
   Clear closet space for equipment
 Second week
   Buy table and stool
   Buy towels, sheets, oil, candles
   Buy filing cabinet
   Get a business phone/fax line
   Get business voice mail
 Third week
   Hang mirror, ceiling fan
   Hang new drapes
 Fourth week
   Convert bathroom for public use

Steps: Advertise/Network
 First week
   Develop a brochure for client mailing
   Make business cards
 Third week
   Visit area health-food stores, chiropractic offices, spas, gyms, or related professions and leave cards and brochures
 Fifth week
   Throw a cocktail party for colleagues, friends, and area merchants
 Seventh week
   Place an ad in local health magazine

Steps: Physical Conditioning/Practice
 First week
   Start and end each day with strengthening and stretching exercises: yoga, fingertip push-ups, crunches, back extension exercises, hand strengthening
 Third week
   Continue strengthening and stretching, add aerobic exercise: fast walking, jogging, biking, swimming

Give one massage every other day
Receive one massage each week
Fifth week
Strengthening/stretching exercises
Give one massage every day
Do one exchange per week (tutorial)
Seventh week
Strengthening/stretching exercises
Give multiple massages per day
Do one exchange per week (tutorial)

This three-part structure—decision making, goal setting, and individual steps—helps you achieve your goals by focusing on a graduated format so as not to become overwhelmed with the process as a whole. It is important to give yourself a time frame so you have a benchmark to evaluate your progress. It is also good to remember that the process is important to setting the tone for your practice and maintaining a healthy state of mind. If you focus on the process, then the product (goal) becomes another delightful and rewarding step in your process and not just a benchmark for success or failure.

You can also use this format to define and outline your short-term and long-term goals in all aspects of your business.

Make a copy of the following page and fill in the individual steps, depending on your goals and resources.

Checklist: Setting Goals

Decision: I want to set up a part-time private practice in my home.

Goal: Physical
Short-term: Work consistently with my nondominant hand
Long-term: Develop the strength to practice massage full-time

Steps: 1.

2.

Goal: Financial
Short-term: Pay back student loans
Long-term: Build client base to support myself through lean times

Steps: 1.

2.

Goal: Educational
Short-term: Review anatomy, physiology, and pathology
Long-term: Study and practice shiatsu

Steps: 1.

2.

Goal: Networking
Short-term: Advertise in local health/trade magazines
Long-term: Develop working relationships with area doctors and massage therapists

Steps: 1.

2.

Remember that with all goals, whether long- or short-term, it is important to outline individual steps to achieve them. Don't forget to write them down, so over time, you can remind yourself of your goals, evaluate your progress, and make adjustments where necessary.

Packaging the Product

If our product is "the work," then we are the package. This may seem silly, but our appearance and demeanor are vitally important to successfully selling ourselves, and by extension our work, to the public. We are trying to convince people that we are skilled, professional, friendly, compassionate, discreet, and clean enough for them to feel comfortable enough to take their clothes off and allow us to touch them. Image is vitally important in our business. We may be the most skilled practitioner on the planet, but if we look or sound anything less than clean, polite, and professional, getting clients will be nothing but difficult. We have to consider our target market.

> One thing that worked in a really small town was taking my personal image and thinking about how I fit into that place. I ended up running around dressed like Mary Tyler Moore for a year, because I was very aware of being a touch therapist in a small town. It worked very well; I got feedback later, after I got to know people, that I didn't look like one of those "strange hippie whatevers."
>
> Mary, Amherst, MA

The world of massage has an allure and an image all its own, which allows a fair amount of latitude when considering appearance. A therapist with long hair or tie-dyed clothing won't raise too many eyebrows in most communities. But if you are trying to sell yourself in a retirement community, piercings, tattoos, and green hair might be a hard sell. These stylistic choices might be an asset, though, if you're targeting a rock 'n' roll band. Since massage crosses all markets, though, do yourself a favor by making your image palatable to as many markets as possible (or at least as many as you are interested in working with).

> I can walk into twenty massage schools, and I will see people
> with their shoes off, piercings, hair dye, whatever. The attitude
> is, "Well that's the profession." But when you leave school, what
> demographic are you going to attract?
>
> Diane, New York, NY

Regardless of stylistic choices, we need to be aware that how we package ourselves is the first step in how we sell ourselves. Above all, we need to be clean and polite. I am always surprised to meet a massage therapist who hasn't considered fingernail hygiene before leaving home. Our hands are the tools of our trade. If you don't make the effort to treat them with care, what sort of message does the potential client receive when shaking hands? Clean, well-manicured hands serve as a billboard (or probably more intimately as a business card) for what you do. We should consider everyone, at every turn during the day, to be a potential client, and before leaving home we should consider every aspect of our appearance and our demeanor. Simple, polite gestures like holding doors for people or offering our seat on a bus can be the conversation starter that leads to a new client.

> Being clear on what it is that you do is really important, and to really
> be a professional, you have to present yourself as one—keeping on
> time, upholding yourself, and upholding the profession.
>
> Denise, San Francisco, CA

Selling yourself invariably involves talking about yourself and your profession. Let me say emphatically when talking about oneself, less is more and listening is better. Selling anything involves communication. Half of communication involves listening, except in massage therapy. Listening is ninety percent of our work, on and off the table.

Regardless of what massage class I am teaching, I introduce my students to the idea of selling themselves in social situations. I give them exercises where they pretend they are at a cocktail party or meeting a friend on the street and get them to practice answering these questions in a simple, concise conversational style:

What do you do?
What is Swedish massage?
Is Swedish massage from Sweden?
What types of massage do you practice?
What is the difference between Swedish massage and shiatsu?
Why should I have a massage?
What are the benefits of massage?
Is chiropractic work good for me?
Do you know a good chiropractor?
What is Reiki? Reflexology? Aromatherapy?
What is the difference between acupuncture and acupressure?

> I think if you are clear about what you want to do, chances are
> that's what will come. Feel the passion that you have for this
> work, and let that come through in the way you talk to people
> and the way you interact with people—that in itself will speed
> the process.
>
> Peggy, Melbourne, FL

> Focus on what you love about the work and learning how to say
> that to people.
>
> Mary, Amherst, MA

Being knowledgeable and articulate about all aspects of your profession
makes you professional in the eyes of a potential client. Knowing
a network of other practitioners in your area implies that you are
established and connected.

> What helped me initially was getting connected with a chiropractor
> and other healing professionals. It's a good thing to be able to
> have a broad referral source for your clients—it helps you seem
> professional, and it helps you help your clients.
>
> Denise, San Francisco, CA

A word of caution: even though someone may ask you a specific question regarding your profession, I guarantee that they are not as interested in the details of massage therapy as you are—so keep your responses concise and entertaining, if possible. Essentially you want to come across as intelligent, knowledgeable, easy-going, interesting, interested, calm, and compassionate. Practice answering any of these questions in fifteen to twenty seconds and then listen. If a potential client is interested in learning more, they will pursue the conversation. Long-winded didactic conversation on any subject is boring and a turn-off and is certainly not a way to win over potential clients.

Advertising

Before you can think about ways to advertise, you need to first define and determine your target market. Your target market is the group of people to whom you want to sell your product or service.

Who is your market?
Essentially you want to determine who in your area will want, need, or can afford massage. Then, of that group, on whom do you want to focus your energy to make them aware of your product? You do not have to exclude any market, but you want to tailor your message for different types of clients. For the athlete client, you might explore road races and talk about the benefits of pre- and post-race sports massage. For the retiree, you could visit retirement facilities and talk about how massage increases circulation and reduces pain. Massage is good for everyone, so essentially your approach is limited only to the ways in which you can think to sell it and yourself.

> You should have a basic idea of how the economy in your area works. Have an idea of who lives there, which people might be interested in getting massage, and whom you have to contact. Is it a tourist-type place? Is there a particular neighborhood or area where there are wealthy people? Is there a school where there is a sports program? Who is going to be interested in getting your work?
> Mary, Amherst, MA

Where is your market?

Next you need to consider where to find your market and tailor your work, your message, and your appearance to appeal to the target client. Sometimes this process is obvious, but sometimes it requires a little creative thinking. The list below is a starting point.

Target Market: Athletes
Road races
Marathons
Triathlons
College sports
Swim meets
Tennis tournaments
Golf tournaments
Bike races
Professional teams

Target Market: Medical Patients
Hospitals
Hospices
Clinics
Doctors' offices
Chiropractic offices
Physical therapy offices
Acupuncture offices

Target Market: Retirees
Community centers
Nursing homes
Assisted-living communities
Retirement communities

Target Market: Businesses
Corporate Human Resources departments
Hotels
Cruise ships
Resorts
Spas

Pilates studios
Health clubs
Health-food stores

Target Market: General
Street fairs
Airports
Shopping malls
Conventions and trade shows
Health fairs
Adult education
Laundromats
Church gatherings
School events
School or church benefits
Charity auctions

How do you get their attention?
Once you have determined the "who" and the "where" of your target market, then you can determine the "how"—how to best get their attention. You can create printed material like business cards or a brochure to leave in public places or even target specific businesses or communities with a direct mailing. You can buy ads in specific publications that share your target market. You can buy TV or radio ads to advertise your product. You can even organize public awareness events or demonstrations to introduce the community to you and to your work." The Internet is an inexpensive and efficient way to advertise products and services directly to the public.

> I put an ad in a monthly newspaper. It's twenty dollars a month, and it has paid for itself all the time I've had it. But it has also been a kind of irritant, because you get some people calling basically for sexual services.
>
> Tony, Denver, CO

In my experience, ads and mailings are the least effective forms of advertising in the massage profession and certainly one of the most expensive. The best way to advertise is to meet prospective clients in person. Any event that brings us face to face with others is a better way to connect with potential clients.

> Most of my clients come from other clients who've gotten good results, and so they tell their friends. One time I sent out letters to physicians, and I don't think I got many responses to that. It's personal contact. I think it's being involved in a community that has really helped.
>
> Peggy, Melbourne, FL

One-on-one advertising

Regardless of the setting (doctor's office, spa, road race) or the target market, the one-on-one approach to advertising is the most effective for your business and for your money. For the most part, people like to see what they are buying or they want to know (from someone they trust) that the service they will receive comes highly recommended. This is the basis of networking. One satisfied customer (client, friend, or colleague) tells a friend and potential client what a wonderfully caring, compassionate, polite, knowledgeable, and skilled therapist they know, and the phone starts ringing. This kind of advertising requires time and patience but generally circumvents questionable or undesirable clients. Before your friends and colleagues will recommend you, though, they need to know your work is worthy of commendation. In addition, you may need to provide them with impetus to recommend your services. You might offer a discounted rate for each referral. A free massage might be too generous, unless the new referral turns into a regular client, in which case the free session is a small investment by comparison. Adding an extra fifteen to thirty minutes to a session is a nice way to show your appreciation with little, if any, downside.

I am also hesitant to suggest free massage because it devalues the work and can psychologically impair your commitment to the free session and your client's perception of your professionalism and success. We never want to seem desperate for clients—people are attracted to successful people and wary of those who are too eager. But promotions, specials, or discounts for getting people into your space and familiar with your work can be a good way of connecting with potential clients. They know where and how you work and have the first-hand experience with which to recommend you to their friends and colleagues.

> I still advertise by word-of-mouth and flyers. I give my clients half-price coupons to give to their friends, and a couple of times a year I run a half-price sale.
>
> Theresa, Seattle, WA

Targeting professionals like doctors, physical therapists, personal trainers, salon owners, or even hairdressers for discounted or introductory sessions is a good idea, because their clients are potential massage clients. Donating a gift certificate for an introductory massage session to a school or church fund-raising auction is another way to deepen your connections to the community and introduce yourself to potential clients.

> When I went into business for myself full-time, I did what I called a community service project around the neighborhood, where I offered a really low introductory rate massage. It was especially for people who worked in the neighborhood, and it worked beautifully. I'm still in that neighborhood, and I still have a relationship with these people, and they still refer other people. The thing about our business is that it is personal, and so the best way to get things going is through hands-on kinds of advertising versus just advertising in a magazine or newspaper. When I say 'hands-on,' I mean walking out, meeting people, handing them something, and developing a relationship.
>
> Denise, San Francisco, CA

Public places and events
Setting up shop or advertising at public places and events (street fairs, sidewalk art shows, church events, charity auctions, conventions, races, walk-a-thons, athletic tournaments) generally requires some authorization or licensing fee from a city, public authority, or event organizer. Beyond that, for most public places, you need only show up with a massage chair, a sign, and a stack of business cards or brochures.

Your presence is your ad. Here again, you need to make sure you package yourself to appeal to the target market and certainly make sure you have the time, patience, and energy to sell yourself and your work in a caring, compassionate, and professional way.

> As I was working at a gym, I took the time and made the effort to get to know the staff and the trainers, and eventually I worked into several reciprocal arrangements where I'd refer clients to a trainer and they referred their client for massage. I worked out at the gym and hung out there some, which allowed me to get to know the clients at the gym and make sure my presence was known—so that they knew there was a massage therapist on duty and felt comfortable booking work with me, because they had talked to me for half an hour on the treadmill.
>
> Theresa, Seattle, WA

Meeting people in this grass-roots way is a great way to appeal to potential clients. It is similar to a politician glad-handing the public to get their votes. The potential client gets a first-hand look and feel for who you are and what you do. It is still a hard sell but is much more personal and effective than a brochure or a flyer. In this environment, though, a well-designed brochure and business card with clear contact information and explanation of services is a vital tool for advertising, especially when you are busy with another client. Sending people home with a written reminder of who you are and what you offer enhances your professional stature while facilitating future communication.

Local businesses
If you are targeting specific businesses in your area, you might start by contacting their human resources department. A massage-school placement service can also be a valuable resource for connecting with local companies.

> I discovered there's a lot of support you can get from your school, not only placement services, but through a network of people you get to know in the industry.
>
> Theresa, Seattle, WA

Draft a letter of introduction and include articles or studies that talk about the benefits of massage in the workplace. If you have a professional letterhead, it will give a more professional appearance. In the letter, mention that you will follow up with a phone call and then try to arrange a meeting or even a demonstration. If you say you will call within a week, follow through. If you want to be treated as a professional, it is vital to act like one. Even if your initial contact is rebuffed, don't forget to maintain a professional demeanor. A rebuff in the business arena could change in a few months, or it may lead to a network of private clients. Either way, you are building the groundwork, a network, for establishing a practice.

Printed Material

Though printed material alone is generally less effective than one-on-one contact in generating new clients, it is nonetheless important to have professional-looking business cards and, if necessary, brochures. There is an art and a science to effective advertising and the graphic arts. It is probably a good idea to seek the advice of a professional. At the very least, before printing large quantities of material, have someone review and edit material for clarity, grammar, and spelling. (Bartering for design services and printed material is common.) Let's explore some different approaches to advertising in print.

Business cards

Business cards are a standard for professionals in any business. They tell people who you are, what you do, and how to get in touch with you. They introduce you and hint at your personality. A colorful card suggests a colorful personality, while a traditional design may suggest a more conservative personality. Cards also serve as a reminder to people that they met you and that they need a massage. Personally, I believe the simpler the design, the better. I can often identify beginning therapists by the large amount of information packed onto their business cards. In an attempt to legitimize their skills, young therapists feel the need to list every massage skill they have studied or practiced. Besides being confusing and hard to read, this projects a sense of insecurity. The basic information—name, occupation, and contact information—is enough. Inclusion of an address may vary, depending on whether you work in an office or at home and how safe you feel advertising your address. At the very least, a phone number and an e-mail address are necessary, as well as your professional website URL, if you have one. "Occupation" could be as simple as including the initials LMT after your name or, to be safe, "Licensed Massage Therapist." Anything beyond this basic information is extraneous.

Some therapists have a bi-fold card or double-sided card that includes room for appointment information. Though such cards are unusual (and in advertising it is the unusual that attracts attention), essentially I think it is a waste of money. Your card is a reminder of you. Regardless of what the card does or looks like, people will keep it based on their impression of the person from whom they received it. A couple of strong suggestions: make sure the font style and size are legible for both young and old eyes. A lovely, flowing font may evoke the lyrical quality of your work and personality, but if your clients have a hard time deciphering the information, you do yourself a huge disservice. Before printing thousands of cards, brochures, or postcards, it's a good idea to show the design to a cross-section of friends and colleagues for feedback. It is amazing how a simple artistic choice can elicit a vast array of unexpected responses.

Brochures

A brochure is essentially an educational tool, an efficient way to communicate a fair amount of specific information in a small amount of space. It informs your potential clients about who you are, what you do, and how to reach you. It is the business card on steroids. This form of advertising can be produced inexpensively on a home computer or more expensively by a printing service. If you do not want to hire a graphic designer, the AMTA, among many other organizations, offers marketing software, templates, and inexpensive preprinted brochures explaining all aspects of massage therapy. In your brochure, you might want to briefly explain who you are, what you do, and perhaps where you were educated and trained. This gives you credibility. Listing the benefits of massage begins to educate prospective clients of the value and importance of massage. All information should in some way relate to the service you are providing (listing your interests and hobbies will make the brochure seem less professional and more like a personals ad). As with the business card, simple is better. Artwork, especially photography, can be particularly helpful, because it shows people what to expect, what you and your space look like. Research has shown that people are more likely to respond to an ad with a picture than one without. Be sure that your photos look professional but not glamorous (this can lead to unwanted inquiries). The overriding idea is to keep all the information organized in a clear and concise way.

Next you can list a menu of services and prices. If there are different charges for different modalities or for different lengths of time, be sure to organize the information so there is no confusion. You may want to print your menu and prices on a separate card or insert so that when your fees change, the brochure is not obsolete.

Finally, list your contact information and hours of operation. This information needs to be printed clearly and in a prominent place (or perhaps more than one place) for easy reference.

> Actually, I would suggest collecting brochures to see what it is that you like. I looked around at what various people did. I liked brochures that had pictures of the therapist, so you could actually see them. I looked at how each therapist spoke about themselves, about their work.
>
> Denise, San Francisco, CA

Before creating a brochure, determine where and how you are going to use it. Determine who your target market is so you can include information that will appeal to them specifically. If you are targeting athletes or dancers, you might include a short section on the benefits of pre- and post-event massage and a blurb on injury rehabilitation. If you work in a chiropractor's office, you might want to include a short paragraph on the benefits massage provides in conjunction with chiropractic adjustments. Testimonials from clients or quotes from medical journals and trade magazines can confer a certain degree of legitimacy for an apprehensive new client.

Direct-mail marketing

For the most part, printed material is far more effective when combined with a one-on-one approach rather than a mass mailing. People are more likely to read the information if there is a person with whom they relate it (for instance, a chiropractor who has recommended your services, or perhaps a potential client you met at a health fair). But if your flyer is going to be used for direct mailing, consider including space for a mailing label, return address, and stamp to eliminate the expense of mailing envelopes. (The post office's website, www.usps. com, outlines requirements for direct mailing.) Direct mailings are best used when targeting specific groups with common interests. A letter of introduction helps to personalize the information for a direct mailing, especially if a follow-up phone call is indicated. Your brochure can also serve to communicate information when posted on a bulletin board that targets a specific market (for instance, in a yoga or dance studio).

Postcards

Postcards are similar to brochures in their approach and function but generally convey less information and are less expensive to produce and to mail. Like any direct mail, postcards need to first get the potential client's attention and then impart the essential information about your business. Postcards are good tools for communicating a feeling or identity by using a carefully designed logo, artwork, or photography. Often one side of the postcard is used for artwork and the other to convey information. The artwork needs to be eye-catching so that the potential client doesn't reflexively discard the card. The side of the postcard with the information should convey information concisely and organized in an easy-to-read format. Again, a visit to the USPS website will help with requirements for mailing. (Oversize and odd size cards require extra postage.) A series of postcards mailed at intervals is a good and relatively inexpensive way to consistently expose potential clients to the availability of your services, advertise specials, or renew old contacts. Holiday cards, birthday cards, and thank-you cards with personalized messages are a good reminder to clients that massage is just a phone call away.

Websites

With the advent of the Internet, a unique, efficient, and inexpensive form of communication and advertising was born. For the entrepreneur, a website is a virtual necessity for advertising one's wares. Armed with a business card that legibly spells your website address, you put all of your business facts and figures at any potential client's fingertips. With minimal computer skills, you can create an inexpensive, basic web page to advertise your business. A web search can provide a list of companies, some free, that provide web page templates. Or you can barter with a professional website designer or computer-savvy friend.

Your website does not have to be fancy, but it should be easy to find the basic information: location, contact info, services offered. The look, as with your business card, is best kept clean and simple.

Press releases

A press release is an announcement to the community at large and especially the media—your local newspapers, magazines, television stations, and Internet sites—regarding your business and the services you provide. It is generally written to announce a new business, a new location, or an expansion of services. When writing a press release, think about whether you can tie your services in with a local story or issue. If so, you are more likely to catch a news editor's eye. Targeting the health, style, or business editor is also a good idea. Along with the press release, you might include a gift certificate so the editor can experience your services firsthand.

Local papers and magazines often feature an annual edition dedicated to spas, yoga studios, personal training, area gyms, or health in general. Timing a news release for this health-related issue could smartly access a new audience. If such a resource doesn't exist in your area, consider researching it and writing it yourself. It is a great way to network and meet like-minded professionals while also advertising your own business. If you are not proficient at writing, you might do the research and hire a writer. A press release needs to be well written and informative in order to capture media attention. It's always a good idea to get a professional editor to review any work before publication.

Articles

An article for a trade magazine or special interest group, a company newsletter, or a community newspaper is a little more specific in its approach and its target audience. Typically, such articles aim to inform or educate readers about a particular subject or condition. First, consider your target audience in order to gauge its vocabulary and general knowledge of the subject. If you are working in a chiropractor's office, for instance, you might consider writing an article on the benefit of massage therapy in conjunction with chiropractic work. If you do on-site work in an office building, you might write an article on the benefit of good ergonomics and massage for treating carpal tunnel syndrome. Keep your article brief, without too many confusing and technical terms. A well-written article can convey a level of professionalism and expertise, and it is a great way of advertising your practice. Don't forget to post your article on your website, too.

Newsletters

Newsletters—whether by e-mail or a postal flyer—can be a professional and personal way to communicate with your clients. You might publish a quarterly or biannual newsletter with brief articles espousing the benefits of massage. You could write about trends in your practice or massage in general and suggest preventative exercises or techniques to complement your massage work. You might also advertise specials and promotions to entice clients to make an appointment. You can highlight other health practices and events (yoga, tai chi, Pilates, a health fair) in your area to help people stay body-conscious and health-minded. I have seen some newsletters that have health-related crossword puzzles, jokes, and cartoons. Certainly the more entertaining and friendly the publication, the more likely it is to be read. Producing a regular newsletter requires a certain amount of planning and dedication but can be a very effective way of communicating with clients and colleagues while advertising your practice to a specific target audience. Even for your current clients, a newsletter reminds the busy client to make an appointment and also helps convey a level of expertise and professionalism so they feel comfortable referring their friends to you.

It can also keep you visible and connected within the health-care community, another networking tool at your disposal.

The Follow-Up Strategy

Salespeople and telemarketers know the value of a good lead over a cold call. This idea can be put to great effect in our business as well. I call it the follow-up strategy. The follow-up has three parts: the Before, the During, and the After. This is something you can use during a massage session or even when meeting a potential new client.

The Before involves listening and registering information about your clients or potential clients. The information you learn in the initial encounter or phone call will inform not only your work but also your approach to each client. If a client is in pain or has tried other modalities with little effect, it is important to hear their frustration and try to address their concerns. By simply listening and acknowledging our clients' concerns, you set them at ease. People don't expect miracles, but they do expect to be heard. In my intake session with a new client, I have developed a very conversational style, with little writing, trying to engage my clients and put them at ease. I ask pertinent questions and mentally register all information, to be notated and filed while they undress and again after the session.

During the session, I refer to the information I learned in the intake not only to let the client know I have heard them but to continue to engage them in the process. Often clients remember vital information once they have relaxed into their sessions.

The After session has two parts: the Immediate After and the Later. The Immediate After revolves mostly around asking, "How do you feel?" Even though a client and I have just shared a massage experience (I encourage them to communicate during our session), I still want to acknowledge that their personal experience, good or bad, is important and of value. Afterward I will often ask if they have any questions, comments, or concerns to provide space for them to talk and for me to listen. We can't listen too much. Many times a client learns or remembers something during the session that could be beneficial for future work. This time also allows me to evaluate my work through the client's experience and continues to inform my choices for the future or for teaching them exercises or stretches that will help them to help themselves.

It is not unusual for clients to be relaxed and unresponsive immediately after a session, so expecting detailed feedback is probably unrealistic. Giving clients permission to contact you with feedback after the session may produce valuable information for future sessions but should be considered carefully. This is crossing a privacy boundary, and you may not want to extend this invitation to all—or any—of your clients. You might wait until getting to know a client well before suggesting this. Another option is to suggest that clients write down questions, changes, or the perceived effects of the work and bring them to their next session. Alerting clients to the effects of the massage (whether they will be sore) and then how to deal with them (stretching, icing, drinking more water, or soaking in a warm salt bath) may prolong the effects of their sessions both physically and psychologically while also empowering them to take responsibility for their own healing.

The Later is a follow-up call a day or two later, inquiring about the after-effects of the massage. This is smart for two reasons. First, it gives us feedback about our work and insight on how to proceed in the future. And second, from a marketing perspective, it sends a message to our clients that we care. The follow-up is primarily about listening and letting our clients know that we hear them. Listening, whether before, during, or after a session is the key to developing a good bedside manner. A good bedside manner is essentially about setting our clients at ease. If we simply take the time to listen to their concerns and take them into consideration from session to session, we will be perceived as caring, compassionate, and professional. This, by itself, is the greatest marketing tool to have. The best and most effective advertising is word-of-mouth. A satisfied customer who sells our work to a friend is both invaluable and inexpensive.

The follow-up has another purpose, which is about reminding your clients that you are available for referrals. There is nothing wrong with asking clients for referrals or sending them a reminder card from time to time. You might, for instance, send a new client a simple thank-you card expressing gratitude for the business and take the opportunity to include an offer for a discount for referrals or for a prepaid package of massages. For established clients, a follow-up card might come in the form of a birthday card or a holiday card with a special discount. These devices are transparently about drumming up business, as they should be; that is their intent. In general, people respect the entrepreneurial spirit, but only if they also respect the person and the work. All correspondence, as with our work, should be highly professional.

Networking

Networking is the oldest and most effective form of business promotion and advertising. Networking is essentially about developing a group of friends, colleagues, acquaintances, and businesses that are familiar with you and your product. The most modern example of networking (though in our business not necessarily the most effective) is the Internet. The Internet casts a wide net and can be extremely effective in advertising to a large number of people with relative ease and little expense. But the most effective way for massage therapists to develop a network of like-minded colleagues and clients is by meeting people directly and developing personal relationships. People generally search for their private practitioners (doctors, dentists, lawyers, massage therapists) through word-of-mouth, not through the Internet or the yellow pages. They want recommendations from friends whose opinions they know and trust.

Talking to people about what you do is the first step to building a network. (Remember, you should sound professional, informed, and articulate, not desperate). Meeting like-minded professionals is a smart way to begin networking. Taking classes or seminars is a great way to meet other health-care professionals. Other networking ideas include:

Checklist: Other Networking Ideas

1. Arrange an open house to promote an introductory offer

2. Join a professional networking group in your area

3. Join a professional networking group on the Internet

4. Register with the Chamber of Commerce

5. Join an area small-business organization

6. Visit area businesses
> Discuss promotional packages
> Promote joint business opportunities

7. Visit area health-food stores
> Take a part-time job there
> Promote a chair massage day

8. Visit area gyms or spas
> Take a part-time job there
> Promote package deals

9. Take a workshop

10. Visit related medical specialists and practitioners:
> Acupuncturists, chiropractors, physiatrists, physical therapists
> Take a full- or part-time job in their office
> Promote package deals or first-time discounts

11. Join a church group or social organization

12. Post material on a community bulletin board

Regardless of which of these approaches you try, remember that massage is an intimate and personal endeavor. In order to be most effective, your networking should also be intimate and personal. Networking does involve selling yourself and your work, but the best selling involves listening and responding to each individual's personal needs.

Other Marketing Considerations

Be competitive

When determining your market, you may have to do a little homework. Start by getting several massages in your area to see what your competition offers and what kind of clients they are serving. You might ask the other clients (without seeming predatory) what they like about the establishment and their services, and ask the therapists (without seeming nosy) what the clients like. Revealing that you are a new therapist in the area may help you get information, but it may also raise competitive eyebrows. This adventure should give you an idea of what the marketplace is offering and help you to determine how your product could be different or better. One important area where you can be competitive is quality of service. How you deliver the service can make all the difference in your client's enjoyment and desire for the service. A gracious, appreciative, compassionate, and accommodating personality sells. Your work may be physical and demanding, but you need to deliver it with a smile and without attitude if you want your clients to come back.

Offer variety

It's a good idea to have variety both in the clients you appeal to and the services you provide, but you must match the services to the clientele. If you are going to offer a new modality that is not offered by other therapists in your area, first make sure the market needs or wants it. Offering pregnancy massage in a retirement community is probably not a good idea. Promoting a new or unfamiliar modality like shiatsu may require first educating your clients. By educating your clients, you develop a professional profile in the community and build stronger relationships. All business is about developing relationships. You might even consider offering a free seminar, workshop, or open house to bring awareness to the community about your presence and your variety of services.

Emphasize convenience and availability
Convenience and availability are major considerations when trying to be competitive. If booking or getting to a session is difficult, clients will go elsewhere. Yet when it comes to massage therapists, a small amount of accommodation can produce a fiercely loyal client.

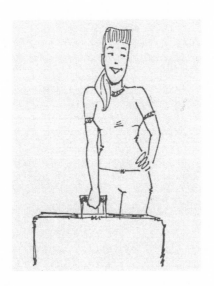

Golden Rule 7

First impressions are the strongest.

Dress to sell yourself.
The first and final touch will linger most.
Give your touch confidence, creativity, variety, and compassion.

8. Interviewing for a Job

Informal Interviews

Not unlike the actor, the massage therapist is always interviewing for the next job. Everyone is a potential employer: people on the street, friends of friends, neighbors, new acquaintances, and other professionals. The interview comes in the form of casual conversation. Talking about your profession in a knowledgeable, articulate, enthusiastic, and friendly way is the best way to sell yourself to a potential client.

> All my work comes from word-of-mouth. Because I'm excited about what I do, I talk about it.
>
> Peggy, Melbourne, FL

As a therapist, regardless of whether you work for yourself or you choose to work for someone else, you are always selling yourself and, by extension, advancing your own career as well as the profile of the profession. Bearing in mind that you can meet new people and impress potential clients anywhere—at a party, at a laundromat or supermarket, or even at the gym—it's a good idea to always carry business cards and dress accordingly. And above all, hygiene should forever be a primary concern: clean clothes, tidy hair, and impeccable fingernails.

Formal Interviews

Interviewing for a therapist position in a more formal setting (spa, hotel, gym, or doctor's office) requires some forethought and preparation beyond appearance, demeanor, and the ability to intelligently and enthusiastically articulate what you do. Most interviews for a massage position have two parts: the conversation and the hands-on component. It should go without saying that your appearance forms the first impression, and that sets the tone for the rest of the interview. Take a moment to consider the establishment where you are interviewing and dress accordingly, bearing in mind that you will probably be giving a massage. Clean, modest, loose-fitting gym wear may be appropriate for an interview at a health club, whereas interviewing at a doctor's office may call for dressing in a more corporate or medical style, like a white shirt and dress pants. Wear a nice T-shirt under the dress shirt for the hands-on component, or carry a change of clothes. If you have an interview at a spa, consider dressing similarly to the therapists who already work there; this gives the interviewer a visual cue that you will fit in. For women, it is a little trickier, because you don't want a work shirt to be too low, too tight, or too revealing. Layering a comfortable work shirt under a dressier blouse for the interview might be a good idea. Unless you live in a tropical climate, wearing shorts, for men or women, is probably too casual, and for women it may be too sexy or suggestive.

Shoes can also be tricky. Balancing the need to perform a massage with the need to present a professional appearance narrows the choices. Wearing a nice pair of gym shoes would not be out of the question, but do be sure they are impeccably clean.

In preparation for working and sweating, it's a good idea to bring a hand towel and a bottle of water. Don't forget to bring a bottle of massage oil or cream and a timepiece to monitor your progress and end on time; this will facilitate your work and create the impression that you are professional and prepared.

Arriving and ending the massage on time is, of course, imperative. Not only is this a professional standard, but it also sends the signal that you are a reliable time manager. During the massage session itself, remember to communicate clearly, ask for guidance and feedback, and adjust your intent accordingly. Listening and checking in throughout the session is a good idea, although talking too much can be annoying.

Conversation cues should be taken from the interviewer, but in general, listening is always better than talking. Bring a few business cards and a current resume, and come prepared with references. Finally, familiarize yourself with the services the establishment offers and come prepared to explain how and why you are a good choice for employment.

Checklist: A Formal Interview

1. Be prompt

2. Dress professionally: hair, nails, shoes, clothes

3. Come prepared:
   Resume
   Business cards
   Timepiece
   Massage cream or oil
   Handkerchief, hand towel, water

4. Communicate concisely and articulately

5. Arrive well rested and enthusiastic

6. Listen and follow instructions

7. Ask for feedback

8. Adjust to client's demands

9. End the massage on time

10. Come prepared with appropriate questions

> I would recommend to anyone going to get a job to interview the person interviewing you. Go in with a list of questions to help you understand if that's where you want to work.
>
> Diane, New York, NY

It is a great idea to interview your interviewer. This may seem odd at first, but besides empowering you, it sends a signal to your potential employer that you are conscientious and serious about your work. It also gives you material for conversation; remember, your interviewer may feel a bit awkward, too, and asking him or her a few questions can break the ice. A friendly and easy conversational style tells the interviewer that you will be friendly and comfortable with customers. Finally, remember that you are interviewing the establishment, too, and you may discover that the job is not right for you. If that is the case, it's better to find out at the beginning.

Come prepared with pencil and paper to take notes for future reference. Questions of basic importance include:

Hours of operation?
Hours of employment?
Flexible schedule?
Responsibilities?
On-call responsibilities?
Extra responsibilities: cleaning, restocking?
Pay? Raises? Tips? Overtime?
Cancellation policy?
Downtime? Breaks? Days off?
Benefits: health insurance, disability?
Continuing education requirements or benefits?
Company policy on sexual advances?
House-call policy?
Noncompete or nonsolicitation policy?

Interviewing for any new job can be scary and uncomfortable. Bear in mind, though, that the interviewer *wants* you to be the perfect fit. An employer wants to hire you so he or she can go about the business of running the business.

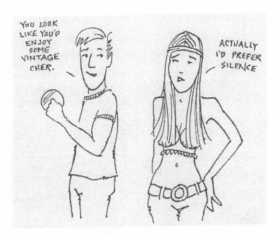

Golden Rule 8

Don't assume anything.

*Ask for direction and give your clients what they
want (within boundaries of course) ...
sound: music/ silence; pressure: light/ deep; tempo: fast/ slow; atmosphere:
light/ dark; candles: scented/ unscented; air conditioning: on/ off.*

9. Boundaries

The single most difficult aspect of massage to fully comprehend, to define, and to clearly articulate in a professional, ethical, and compassionate way is the concept of boundaries.

The very basis of Eastern philosophy is defined by the differentiation of yin and yang, a concept that arose from observing the universe and defining qualities like light and dark, hot and cold, or night and day. Similarly, in early childhood development, concepts like you and me or here and there are the beginnings of differentiation and socialization. All of these concepts allude to boundaries—boundaries are infused in every aspect of our lives.

Likewise, every single aspect of massage, whether physical, social, psychological, sexual, or even financial, is defined by boundaries. Our skill in first defining boundaries for ourselves and then articulating them for our clients will inform not only how we structure our practice but also our professional stature in the community.

Physical Boundaries

Our skin may seem to be our most obvious physical boundary, dividing "self" from "other"—but even that is not as obvious as it first appears. For instance, the area immediately surrounding the body, our "personal space," could easily be considered an extension of the self, but everyone's personal space is different. For instance, someone who lives in a rural environment with large spaces between neighbors might require more personal space than a city dweller. This is a clear example of how boundaries (and not just physical ones) are different for everyone, informed by each individual's experiences and belief system.

The successful therapist needs to recognize and respect the different boundaries and needs that each client brings to the relationship. (Of course, there are certain boundaries that should never be crossed. The most obvious are sexual boundaries, which I'll discuss later in this chapter.) Our clients also need to respect our boundaries in order for our relationship to work, which means that *we* need to articulate *our* boundaries in a clear and compassionate way. The way we communicate our boundaries begins with defining them for ourselves. Our boundaries are infused in every aspect of our behavior at every turn. Uncertainty or even lack of awareness of our own boundaries can easily convey the wrong intention.

Countless scientific studies expound on the necessity of touch to our physical development and well-being, but social and religious mores are often restrictive. It is no wonder that our collective conscious is a little confused in defining appropriate boundaries regarding touch. And each client brings with him a different boundary for appropriate touch. The handshake or the hug as a greeting illustrates different levels of comfort one might have with touch. The therapist and the client each bring their own information, experiences, and issues regarding appropriate touch to their relationship, but it is the therapist who is the professional and therefore the one who is responsible for defining, articulating, and enforcing the boundaries. For example, offering your hand in greeting sets a more formal boundary than a hug or a kiss on the cheek. For some therapists, it is imperative to create and maintain a formal relationship with their clients, and so the handshake feels appropriate. For other therapists, the hug or the kiss on the cheek, especially for long-term clients, seems more appropriate. Offering a hand to a client with whom a relationship has developed for years might be perceived as an insult.

In business relationships you want your clients to feel comfortable. You want them to trust you. They want you to be able to relate to them. Understanding their customs and boundaries helps strengthen your relationship. Diplomats spend hours researching and practicing the local customs of the dignitaries with whom they seek a relationship. To accommodate others, boundaries are crossed and redefined every day. But in order to be comfortable redefining a boundary to incorporate someone else's, you must first be clear about your own.

In defining your boundaries, there must always be a threshold across which you know you will never go. (For example, "I will not have sex with my clients!") This does two things: it creates a sense of security and authority out of which you act and respond to your clients and it communicates on a conscious and subconscious level what your intentions are and are not. People can be clever and unconscious of their needs and desires and seek to have them met in both appropriate and inappropriate ways. Navigating through these "mind"-fields means recognizing the warning signals that can lead to boundary crossing. This is where a course in ethics and boundaries is indispensable and why such courses are offered in massage schools more and more.

Going back to the example of the hug—there are hugs and there are *hugs*. For the therapist where the hug falls within the threshold of acceptable behavior, the hug dilemma—"Was that hug too long or too tight?"—may create uncertainty for both the client and the therapist, depending on the underlying intention. This is where clear personal intention and identification of boundaries followed (when necessary) by articulation helps to defuse an uncomfortable situation. It may also require redefinition of a more cautious boundary. Offering a hand in place of a hug would be a more subtle articulation of a boundary. (Sometimes, though, a definitive, unmistakable, and outright declaration might be required, like: "I do not have sex with my clients." Or, "The happy ending you can expect is in no way sexual. If that is what you are looking for, you need to go someplace else.")

We may think we are creating obvious physical boundaries only to be betrayed by unconscious behavior. We all go through life with conflicts of interest. We may find our clients physically attractive, even though we desire to maintain a strictly professional relationship with them. The very nature of our work crosses normal social boundaries. So defining and maintaining different boundaries can be both confusing and difficult while all the while trying to build a comfortable, compassionate, and professional business relationship.

> Before I was married, I developed a friendship with a client whom I was very attracted to. It was good for me, because I learned the dangers of allowing it to go that way. We were very flirtatious. It's too easy. It's a weird situation. Someone's feeling nurtured; you're feeling appreciated. I realized that if I'm attracted to someone, that's okay; just admit it and put it away. Don't have that as something you can toy with during a massage session. It's okay, that stomach is very pleasing, and go on.
>
> Tamara, Chicago, IL

Social Boundaries

There are tomes of information and research about different societies and social boundaries spanning the ages. The most important thing for a massage therapist to recognize is that socialization can be quite different for each of us, whether we are from across the globe or from across town. If we subscribe to the idea that business is about developing relationships with people, then we must also stay open to the different social customs and mores of our clients. I often suggest to my students that they "stay open to all possibility." By staying open we may be educated or even enlightened.

Notice that I do not say we must "adopt" our clients' customs. A relationship is a dance with two partners. If one partner is constantly stepping on the other's toes, not only is the dance awkward, but it may also be painful. The relationship will not persevere. A criterion or boundary for accepting a good dance partner might be one who dances on the bottoms of their feet and not on the tops of ours. Even if we are open to new ways of thinking, we must be clear about what our parameters for acceptable or, more accurately, unacceptable behavior are.

For example, in some social groups, drinking alcohol is a normal and accepted way of socializing. If one drinks with a business partner or sits down for a meal with her, it is implied that a greater bond of trust is established. In some business circles, if a client offers an alcoholic drink, it would be perceived as rude to decline. But as massage therapists, we would never accept an alcoholic beverage from a client, especially before work, as it is unethical. So if we arrive for a house call and a client offers a drink or even a meal before working, it would be inappropriate to accept, because it would cross an ethical boundary. It is incumbent upon us to decline in a way that defines our ethical responsibility without offending the client's social norm.

Time as a Boundary

From a business perspective, it could be said that a massage session is about selling time. An hour of time is sold for an agreed-upon price. In the (informal) contract, the client expects to receive an hour-long massage (although many spas advertise an "hour" massage when the client really receives a fifty- or fifty-five-minute massage). The hour constitutes a boundary, so anything less than an hour crosses a boundary of accepted or acceptable professional behavior. We could also argue that a session lasting longer than an hour also crosses a boundary. Some clients may be happy to get more time for their money, but the time a client allots for a massage session is based on the time that the therapist or spa advertises. If you go overtime, not only have you broken the contract and created a sense of unpredictability for the client, but you also run the risk of forcing the client to rush to his next appointment, possibly undoing the relaxing effects of his massage. You may thus unintentionally irritate or even alienate the client. If you consistently run overtime and the client starts to expect a longer session, then you have inadvertently set a new time boundary, and ending a future session on time may be perceived as breaking this new, unintentional boundary.

> An hour massage is sixty minutes. For me, it's a matter of pacing. Keeping sessions consistent helps with that. If you don't pace yourself, you quickly become exhausted; then you are more prone to injury, and it can fuzz your boundaries.
>
> Theresa, Seattle, WA

> One way to stay within a particular time boundary is being judicious about the amount of input. Part of that is the attitude, "I don't have to do it all." I am one step in this person's healing journey. Sometimes I get to do the last piece. Sometimes it's my job to teach them to breathe. It doesn't really matter where I am in the journey; I just do my little part.
>
> Peggy, Melbourne, FL

Another way to honor a time boundary is by showing up for an appointment on time. The appointment is a contract between the therapist and the client. There is an acceptable time limit on either side of the appointed time for both people to arrive.

If a client is late, many therapists or spas simply deduct time from the allotted massage session. If the schedule allows little time between sessions, then this deduction becomes necessary to keep from infringing on the next appointment. There is little compassion in this approach, as time and money seem to drive this scheduling arrangement. It also takes what is traditionally seen as a relaxing experience and makes it a rushed or even anxious one for both the client and the therapist. Rushing a client out for the next appointment betrays the compassion he seeks and may injure the relationship. Certainly you should not accept responsibility for tardy clients, but ideally you might build in extra time between appointments to allow for occasional lateness and to help keep the experience as relaxing as possible.

It goes without saying that the therapist, too, is responsible for being on time. Many of us are unhappily familiar with the waiting rooms of our doctor's offices. Not only do we want our practitioners to be present and compassionate to our needs, we also want them to be on time. Whether traveling between appointments or scheduling appropriately, allot ample time between clients to allow for beginning and ending your appointments as contracted. Arriving too early or too late is a boundary infringement (though arriving a few minutes early is better than arriving a few minutes late).

Another time boundary to consider is when not to work. The beginning therapist, struggling to start a practice and attract new clients, is invariably faced with the decision of when and when not to accept a massage request. Especially for the therapist striking out on her own who is striving to build a committed client base, saying no to a willing client can be agonizing. In any customer-service-oriented business, availability is paramount to success. But before we talk about breaking the rules, let's explain why we need a time boundary like this. Burnout is a very real and potentially career-ending phenomenon (see chapter 10, Self-Care). The beginning therapist, striving to grow a fledgling practice, almost begs to have that problem. But it is important to begin running your business so that you consider the factory worker and not just the profit line. Massage work taxes not just the physical body but the mind and the spirit as well. It requires a tremendous amount of energy, discipline, and determination. We need to marshal a vast array of our talents—physical, energetic, and intuitive—to successfully and repeatedly meet the challenges our clients present to us. We need to make sure we refuel the tanks from time to time so that we can come to the work with renewed vigor and vitality for each client and for each massage. Establishing time boundaries for ourselves is vital to maintaining a healthy practice. Taking time off between clients and days off to do nothing is a vital tool for maintaining the reserves needed for our work. A regular day or days off or time off between clients also sets a good example for our clients. Most clients understand the need for downtime—it is usually one of the reasons they are coming to see us in the first place. It is a good idea to simply tell a client who requests a massage on your downtime that you are not available because it is your time off. If they don't understand, then you probably need to reconsider them as a client anyway.

Having said that it is important to set boundaries around when you are available to work, it can also be a relationship-building tool if you are, within reason, flexible to your clients' needs. The key is knowing when to say no. If a regular client has a scheduling problem and you make a compromise, whether it is for their benefit or yours, you cannot resent them for your decision. It is a good idea, though, to let them know that you are making an exception. Remember, though, that this time-boundary compromise should be the occasional exception to the boundary rule; otherwise there is no rule.

In the beginning, I didn't have limitations. I would take a client anytime, anywhere, just so I could make some money. Now I have very specific time restrictions about when I will not work. It's not only knowing what you can and can't do, it's also what you want. Sometimes I just don't want to work on the weekend; I just don't. There is no question in my mind that I have set those boundaries.

Alexis, Wainscott, NY

Payment as a Boundary

Money can be an emotional issue. Setting clear boundaries about how you are paid is imperative for the success of your practice and the health of the relationships with your clients. What and how you are paid is a fundamental aspect of the contract into which you enter with your clients. Setting a fee is setting a boundary. You will provide a massage for a certain amount of money, no less. This boundary seems clear, but it can easily become complicated when you make exceptions for certain groups of people or work on a sliding scale to include "economically challenged" clients. Everyone wants a bargain and everyone wants to feel special. If you are an independent contractor (as opposed to an employee of a spa or massage establishment) people are much more likely to negotiate or even barter for your fee. The client who wants to negotiate can cause a certain amount of consternation for the beginning therapist trying to build a practice. Weighing the loss of a client against working for less can be confusing (see chapter 6, Pricing). This is where you need to be clear and articulate about what is acceptable recompense for your services. Setting a boundary and honoring it is a way of honoring your work, your clients, and yourself. You honor your work and yourself by giving them value. You honor your clients by defining your worth and by being clear and consistent in how you administer your services. There are always exceptions to a rule, but if there are too many exceptions then there is no rule.

The best time to elucidate how you want to be paid (check, cash, credit card) is when making the first appointment. In effect, you are laying out the terms of your contract with your new client. You are setting a boundary. You also need to consider what the consequences are for crossing this boundary or breaking the contract.

> A lot of it has to do with worrying about how people think about me. Do they like my massage? You think, I really need the money, but I don't want to ask them for more money because I want them to ask me back. Nowadays, if someone doesn't want to pay me a certain amount of money, then I won't do it. You have an option. In the beginning you don't see that. You're eager, you're frightened, and you don't have experience. You go through all that insecurity, as you would in any business.
>
> Alexis, Wainscott, NY

The Cancellation Fee

The most contentious aspect of payment is probably the cancellation fee. Many health-care professionals charge a twenty-four-hour cancellation fee to keep clients or patients from canceling at the last minute. Some therapists define a forty-eight-hour cancellation fee as the standard boundary. This presumably allows the practitioner to fill the time slot so there is no lost income. This policy needs to be articulated at the outset of the contract or at the time the initial appointment is made.

In my experience with other health-care professionals, the cancellation fee is articulated and enforced with varying degrees of regularity. For psychotherapists, there seems to be a strict adherence to the cancellation boundary, and most patients accept this. Many medical doctors post the policy at their reception desks without ever verbally announcing the policy. But for massage therapists, regardless of whether the cancellation policy is defined and well articulated, enforcing the policy can be, at the least, an uncomfortable situation. Most long-standing therapist-client relationships develop beyond strict, formal, professional relationships. Ideally, consistency is the best policy, though there may be exceptions that help to navigate through this issue. For instance, there may be a first-time exception to the rule. This allows the therapist to re-articulate the policy, explaining compassionately that when someone cancels at the last minute, we are not compensated for the lost appointment, and it also prevents another client from having that appointment. However, if a client cancels because of illness or because of an emergency, we may reconsider enforcing the policy. Showing compassion for the plight of our clients helps to strengthen our relationship. Some therapists print their cancellation policy on their cards, while others announce their policy on their voice mail or answering machines. Of course, there is no one answer to address this issue. Each client will respond differently to the policy, and so beyond treating each client with compassion, we will always need to weigh the possibility of offending a client against dealing with a habitual boundary crosser. Adhering to the policy and losing a client, in some cases, may be a good idea. The strife and anxiety created from a habitual boundary crosser may not be worth the income they provide. There are varying degrees of tolerance for each client, depending on the strength of each relationship.

Dual Relationships

A dual relationship is when we develop a second relationship with a client in addition to the client/therapist relationship. This might be a client who becomes a friend, or conversely, it could be a family member or colleague who becomes a client. A dual relationship complicates the dynamics between two individuals, because as their roles change, so do the power differentials between them. In addition, issues of transference and countertransference (see Transference and Countertransference, later in this chapter) can complicate and confuse the relationships as individuals shift in and out of their different roles.

We treat a friend differently than a business associate. A family member takes liberties that a client never would. It is not uncommon for a client to feel affection toward a therapist because of the empathetic nature of the therapeutic relationship. It is only a small step for both the client and the therapist to want to expand the professional relationship into a more personal one. This is generally unwise, because the professional relationship does not have the varied dynamics of a friendship. A potential problem with expanding the professional relationship is that the initial relationship may have fostered in the client feelings of gratitude and even adoration for the therapist; the therapist, for his part, may have feelings of grandiosity or something like a God complex. When the relationship changes and the power differential shifts, this can lead to feelings of disappointment, loss, or even anger, when the therapist or client as a friend no longer lives up to the other's idea of what their role should be. Before expanding a professional relationship to include a second type of relationship, it is important to try to evaluate objectively and consider whether your client has an unduly optimistic opinion of you that is either unhealthy or unsustainable. Try to objectively evaluate and determine your own motives for expanding the relationship. Operating from a client-centered model, you might simply ask yourself if the change would be good for the client. If you determine that either of you is not mature enough to handle the added responsibilities of the new relationship, don't do it. If in doubt, you might confer with a colleague or even a mental-health professional. Talking through your concerns with an objective third party may help you to understand your motives and determine if they are healthy for you and especially for your client. Even for the most objective person, the excitement of a new friendship can mask a more dubious motive. In the end, it is better to keep one relationship healthy rather than lose or diminish both.

Friendship as a Boundary

"Don't mix business with pleasure." In general, this is a good rule of thumb. Nonetheless, in practice, especially for therapists who have been practicing with the same clients for years, the social barrier may become permeable over time. Certainly there are some professions where socializing with clients is forbidden—psychotherapy, for example. But there are plenty of other health-care professionals and other professionals (doctors and lawyers, for instance) who commonly foster social relationships with their clients and patients. Without getting into the ethical question of "Is it proper?" we might first ask, "Is it smart?" I don't think there is a right or wrong answer to either question. The answer is different for each individual. For some therapists, keeping a distinct separation between clients and friends is important and a smart idea. This arrangement keeps the relationship on a more simple footing with less opportunity for crossing other boundaries and fluctuating power differential dynamics (see Psychological Boundaries, later in this chapter).

> I went through a period where I realized the work is significantly deep, not just touching the body but also the psyche. So what I discovered through my process was, I don't develop friendships with clients. It is something that I actively practice, to keep the boundary clear and keep clear what our work is about. I find the objectivity and the neutrality needs to be honored.
>
> Denise, San Francisco, CA

On the other hand, showing interest in our clients' endeavors may be smart both politically and economically, and it may also provide inspiration, entertainment, or depth to our professional relationship with them. Entering into a friendship with a client shifts the power differential and forever alters the relationship. The difficult part about this kind of dual relationship is maintaining the professional relationship at the highest level and keeping the two relationships in their proper perspective. (It is probably wise to treat the professional relationship with greater care and professionalism to help define for both you and the client the difference in the two relationships—no shortcuts, cocktails, or relaxed attitude toward the quality of the work.) There is also the added difficulty of whether you will be able to maintain the professional relationship if the friendship comes to an end, or vice versa.

Family Boundaries

Business associates, like family members, require a certain degree of understanding and compromise in order for the relationship to work. Friends and family members don't necessarily make the best business associates, because each has different boundaries for appropriate behavior. Adding a massage relationship to a familial relationship may be a boundary-management nightmare. Dual relationships can be difficult to manage and require a certain degree of maturity and introspection. We also need to consider that altering or ending a dual relationship can severely tax the primary relationship, if not end it.

I had a client who was a friend first, and issues started coming up between us. I didn't feel I could bring up our friendship issues because she was coming to me as a massage therapist, and I started to feel resentful. Similar things started to happen with my family. With family and friends it just gets muddled, because it is a dual relationship. So I start not being able to do things or say things, and they get hurt, and it affects the professional relationship. It gets messy once you go outside the parameters of a professional relationship.

Denise, San Francisco, CA

Psychological Boundaries: The Power Differential

Psychological boundaries require a deep examination that goes beyond the scope of this book. Most comprehensive massage programs offer classes that examine these issues and begin to empower therapists to handle them. Probably the most important psychological dynamic to explore is the power differential.

Massage by nature is a social relationship. There is an inherent social hierarchy. The therapist is the professional, the expert, or perhaps by contrast, the employee; while the client is the recipient, the student, the employer. In each case, one person has a more powerful position. This power differential, in the healthiest of circumstances, creates a relationship where the more powerful person brings benefit to the less powerful. At different moments, each person wields the power: the therapist as he stands over the recumbent client and the client when he assumes the role of employer. The client is vulnerable because he is unclothed (though draped) while the practitioner positions himself within the client's personal space. The practitioner is vulnerable because he seeks the client's approval for future employment. Boundaries keep the power differential of the relationship healthy for both parties. Another, more Eastern approach might be for the practitioner to surrender all claims to power by acknowledging the client as a gift and an opportunity to practice his craft. (This point of view discounts, however, the power of the practitioner's knowledge and experience to help the client.) But even when we attempt to eschew the power position with a client, the health of the relationship demands clearly articulated boundaries.

In the field of massage, where nudity and touch are involved, the influence of psychology infuses every aspect of behavior for both the client and the therapist. The nature of massage crosses normal social boundaries, and so all aspects of behavior, some subtle and some not so subtle, need to be redefined. We are all unique individuals with unique backgrounds and upbringings, and the introduction of touch and nudity may cause a range of responses, both conscious and unconscious. Uncommon situations or experiences can elicit uncommon reactions. As therapists, we need to understand the unusual nature of massage and prepare ourselves for our clients' (and our own) unique responses to our work. Without even examining devious characters with devious intentions, we will encounter a vast array of psychological responses to both our work and ourselves.

> Sometimes I think when people come to see you, they're not even certain of the responses they're having. It probably ignites so much that you can't be freaked out if they go, "Oh, I might be attracted to you, or I might be this," because it's so vulnerable to be touched and have all of someone's attention on you for at least an hour. It just starts everything going.
>
> Tamara, Chicago, IL

Innuendo and humor, especially coming from a first-time client, are ways of psychologically testing the boundaries of this new and unusual relationship. Gently joking about nudity during a massage session may provide a first-time client an outlet to alleviate discomfort, but as with anything, the joke is informed by the underlying intention. How we deal with the joke or innuendo is fully informed by how clearly we have defined our boundaries. This is a good opportunity to articulate them. But bear in mind that using a chainsaw to cut through paper might be an overreaction to the task at hand and may actually indicate a response involving issues of countertransference (see Transference and Countertransference, later in this chapter). We don't want to offend or alienate a client, even if he is fishing. The more secure we are with our boundaries, the less emphatic we need to be in defining them. Our clients may also be testing our boundaries, not necessarily so they can cross them, but so they can relax, knowing we won't cross theirs. Knowing what to expect can be liberating and set some clients at ease, enabling them to relax and enjoy the work even more.

As professionals, we are responsible for defining and maintaining clear boundaries so that we create a safe environment for our clients to receive the work we provide. Therapeutic touch can unlock a plethora of physiological and psychological responses in the body, both conscious and unconscious. When touch elicits strong emotional responses like anger, fear, grief, worry, or even joy, the psychological reaction to this exposure can be unsettling for the client and the therapist alike. A compassionate approach is a good first response to what may appear to be a psychological boundary issue. If the issue persists, a clear articulation of boundaries should follow.

Sexual Boundaries

Before we set a sexual boundary, we need to understand why it is important to have one. Sex is a very normal physiological human need. The study of sexual behavior across many species informs us of complex rituals and behavior that involve dominance and submission in the form of role-playing in order to arouse and stimulate the partners in preparation for the act of sexual relations. Role-playing suggests a set of rules or boundaries, whether innate or imposed. In other words, sex is a very complicated endeavor involving complex physiological and psychological concepts and behavior patterns with roles and rules and reactions, the study of which employs scientists, therapists, behaviorists, ethicists, educators, religious leaders, and even a lawyer or two. With legions of professionals studying, regulating, and enforcing the complicated primal nature of sex and behavior and its effects on society, why not set a boundary for your massage practice that eliminates sex and all the psychological, ethical, and legal baggage that comes with it?

When I have someone on the table that I am attracted to, I deal with it by acknowledging it to myself, not the client. I acknowledge the attraction within myself and just know that it's there and just put it on the shelf, acknowledging it but not acting on it. Once you're aware of it, it makes it a little easier not to let it run the show. It comes back to really knowing yourself. The key things that need to be addressed are your own sexual issues and boundaries. It is really important to know why you're giving somebody your card and where you stand on your own sexual issues and boundaries. How do you say no, especially women? How do you set a boundary? Are you comfortable with it? And if you're not, look at the issue within yourself. The other thing is to really tune into your own intuition. If somebody calls and something is not feeling right, give yourself permission to refer them out.

Denise, San Francisco, CA

If we examine another profession that involves touch and nudity, prostitution (in some minds closely related to massage), we can see how the psychological relationship in our profession can easily become confused and uncomfortable. Nudity and touch, regardless of the profession involved, elicit sexual subtext, whether intentional or unintentional. It is our job as professional massage therapists to inform ourselves of the sexual response that massage can elicit in our clients and ourselves and define and articulate clear, ethical, safe, and compassionate boundaries for dealing with it.

I realized that if I'm attracted to someone, that's okay; just admit it and put it away. Don't toy with it during a massage session. If someone is a little flirtatious, it just doesn't bother me. My husband jokes with me about it. He says, "You do realize you go into a room with someone who's naked, and you touch them for an hour. It is an unusual circumstance for our culture."

Tamara, Chicago, IL

Let me be clear. A compassionate sexual boundary is not one where we acknowledge the build-up of sexual tension with a client so that we compassionately "release" it for them. Massage can easily elicit sexual arousal both for the client and the therapist—there is nothing abnormal about this. A compassionate response to this sexual response might simply be to ignore it rather than "punish" a client for it. I have heard therapists react to clients' arousal with vehemence, as though the arousal were a personal affront to their professionalism. There seems to be a great deal of subtext (countertransference) in such a strong response to what we (should) know is a perfectly natural physiological response to touch. In short, we can't bring our personal issues into the massage room.

I had one male client at a hotel who asked me if massage helped men keep an erection. This is kind of a red-flag question, but I didn't get the sense that it was a come-on. I asked him a couple questions about his health and discovered that he'd just started blood pressure medication. Because I was a stranger, thousands of miles away from home, he felt safe in asking a very personal and, to him, a very frightening question. Another man halfway through his session began apologizing because he had an erection. I explained to him the physiological responses to massage that sometimes occur. He immediately felt better (and his erection went away, because he stopped being nervous). I think therapists who immediately jump all over a client or shame them when they ask questions do themselves and their client a lot of potential harm.

Theresa, Seattle, WA

It is vitally important to clearly define our sexual boundaries before we ever approach the massage room. Whether we fall on the side of the argument that oral sex does not constitute sexual relations, in the world of massage, it most certainly crosses an appropriate boundary into the world of inappropriate sexual behavior. If we acknowledge that sexual subtext, and even sexual arousal, can be a normal response to massage, then we have to fortify ourselves with a nonnegotiable boundary from engaging in any sexual behavior or activity. This commitment protects us and our clients.

> There are so many proactive ways to avoid sexual harassment. You have to go into this with your eyes open. We're in a field of body touching. If you're going to be immature, then you can't be in the field. It's just a hard line. Draw the line. I think nowadays that if your client is inappropriate, there's much more support for you to say, stop. But I really believe it has to come from the therapist.
>
> Diane, New York, NY

Once a professional relationship turns into a sexual one, the power differential shifts and the relationship is changed forever. The professional relationship is sacrificed for a personal one, and a whole new area of behavior is available to both the therapist and the client, whether desired or not. The act of crossing the professional boundary opens the door to an array of nonprofessional or perhaps even unethical behaviors. This in turn may lead to consequences that not only threaten the professional relationship but also, because of the shift in the power differential, could lead to blackmail or, more forthrightly, a lawsuit.

In the classroom, I ask my students to consider this question: "If you have spent all the time, effort, and money to learn to be a professional massage therapist, why jeopardize your reputation and license for sex?" If the desire for a personal relationship with a client overrides the desire for a professional one, then end the professional relationship *before* engaging in a personal one.

> Over the years, I've gotten a lot clearer on knowing what the signals are, and what people are looking for—something more of a sexual nature than a therapeutic nature—and being able to separate that out. At the beginning, it comes back to trusting your gut, really listening to what people are asking for, what they're looking for, especially men to women or women to men. I often just outright ask, "What are you hoping to get from massage?"
>
> Denise, San Francisco, CA

To summarize: Sex is innate. Sex is complicated. Touch may elicit a sexual response. Keep it simple. Don't go there. If you can't help yourself, end the professional relationship first.

> The **NCBTMB Code of Ethics** states that massage therapists should "refrain under all circumstances, from initiating or engaging in any sexual conduct, sexual activities, or sexualizing behavior involving a client, even if the client attempts to sexualize the relationship."
>
> The **NCBTMB Standards of Practice** states that massage therapists should "refrain from participating in a sexual relationship or sexual conduct with a client, whether consensual or otherwise, from the beginning of the client/therapist relationship and for a minimum of six months after the termination of the client/therapist relationship."

Transference

Issues of transference and countertransference are formidable in our profession. They take a great deal of discipline and training both to recognize and to deal with in a healthy, balanced, and compassionate way. These issues are emotional and reactive in nature, and therefore they are often subconscious, buried beneath our ability to reason. The NCBTMB defines transference as "the displacement or transfer of feelings, thoughts, and behaviors originally related to a significant person, such as a parent, onto someone else, such as a massage therapist (or doctor, psychotherapist, teacher, spiritual advisor, etc.)." In our profession, the massage therapist, being in a power position and a position of authority, is often the catalyst and target of these feelings. Because of the intimate nature of massage involving touch and nudity, clients often associate the emotional feelings that are unearthed during massage with past experiences or people who have elicited similar responses in them. These responses, though often negative, can also seem positive. Regardless, both forms are unhealthy, primarily because the client is reacting to something or someone from their past and not to what is actually happening in the present.

A positive transference reaction might be when a client transfers undue praise, authority, or status on the therapist in the process sublimating their deeper feelings. For example, a client may sublimate feelings of discomfort or unhappiness with some aspect of their massage out of respect or reverence for the therapist. As practitioners, we need to be aware of the subtle nature of transference issues and work hard at recognizing the signs that can lead to dysfunctional behavior in our clients and in our reaction to them. Most especially, we should never try to take advantage of a client's transference, even when this falls in the positive and seemingly innocuous realm. For example, it is probably a bad idea to accept an invitation or free tickets to an event from a client whom we suspect has a crush on us.

Transference issues that are negative are probably more easily recognized. Negative transference issues are generally more charged and elicit a stronger emotional reaction from the client. Often the client is reacting to something from their past that makes them feel unsafe or not in control. The power differential between a therapist and the client can trigger feelings of inadequacy or powerlessness, where the client exhibits behavior that questions trust and security. For example, a client who was physically abused as a child may keep her eyes open throughout the massage or try to control the therapist by directing where and how the therapist works. Dealing with negative transference issues can be much more difficult, because our client's behavior is directed at us in a negative and often magnified way. It takes awareness and a degree of training to recognize and effectively deal with these issues as they arise. The most difficult part is not to take transference personally, as this may lead to countertransference issues. Defining and articulating clear boundaries of behavior both inside and outside the massage room are imperative to navigating through these issues both for our own health and well-being and our client's.

Countertransference

Transference and countertransference are not unusual in our profession, and we all deal with them on a daily basis in our practices and in our daily lives. The key to managing these complex psychological dynamics is first to be aware that they exist. It is always a good idea to find a colleague or mental-health professional with whom you can confer to help you navigate through these issues.

The NCBTMB defines countertransference as "a practitioner's unresolved feelings and issues, which are unconsciously transferred to the client." Essentially, countertransference is transference in reverse. The practitioner unconsciously reacts to the client's behavior from some past experience and transfers his feelings from the past onto the current relationship with the client. For example, a therapist who was abandoned by her father may transfer her feelings of anger and resentment onto an older male client who stopped seeing her because his reasons for receiving massage were resolved. In this case, the therapist is reacting to a slight from the past that had nothing to do with the current reality.

In general, we shouldn't expect anything from our clients beyond payment for our services and a certain degree of respect and observance of our implicit and explicit boundaries. We probably should not even expect any tangible results, lest we end up feeling disappointed if we are unsuccessful, therefore transferring those feelings onto our client. That is not to say that we should not have a clearly defined intention with our work, only that it is our client's choice to change or not. We are their facilitators, not their healers. We are all healers, but only to ourselves.

Countertransference can also take the form of both positive and negative reactions to our clients. Strong feelings in any form may be a red flag worth investigating. Feelings, whether good or bad, that elicit an unusual reaction, decision, or response are signs that you are venturing into countertransference territory. For example, do you consistently forgive a chronically late client? Do you dress differently for a certain client? Do you work on a day off or work overtime to accommodate a certain client? Does a certain client elicit ambiguous feelings of affection that alter your usual professional behavior? If the answer to any of these questions is yes, at the very least you should examine your choices and behavior regarding this client and perhaps even seek guidance or feedback from another colleague or professional. If you find that you are hesitant to divulge this altered behavior, out of fear of disclosure or some other emotional reaction, you are probably firmly embedded in a countertransference episode. Keeping the client safe and maintaining a client-centered practice should be your priority. Referring your client to another practitioner is a good first step while you work through the complex dynamics involved.

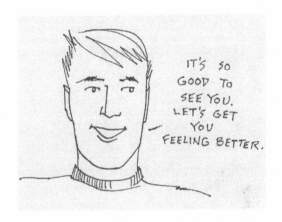

Golden Rule 9

Keep it warm.

Warm hands, warm room, warm disposition.

10. Self-Care

It would be shortsighted to explore the path to a successful career in massage therapy without also discussing self-care. Though there are no comprehensive statistics, I strongly suspect that many massage careers are cut short by injury and burnout (see Burnout, later in this chapter) from overwork and improper body mechanics. In every class I teach, whether beginner or advanced, shiatsu or Swedish, my strongest emphasis is on good body mechanics.

> If ten is most important, body mechanics is around a seven or eight. I'm in this for the long haul, so I have to find a way of doing this so that I don't hurt myself. I might be tired at the end of the day, but I haven't overused. It doesn't make any sense to hurt myself to help someone else. So we need a win-win way to do things, and I like finding unique ways of doing things. If it hurts me, then I have to find another way of doing it so it doesn't hurt.
>
> Peggy, Melbourne, FL

Any repetitive physical endeavor over time will reveal overstressed and weak body parts. Pain is one of our greatest teachers. It tells us that something is wrong and suggests, not so subtly, our need to explore a new way of working.

> In general, I think because I teach massage, I am much more aware of body mechanics. It's part of my everyday life. I try to instill that in my students: "I don't know who taught you that stroke, but if it's hurting you, it's wrong. It might be a great stroke, just wrong for you. Let's find another way of doing it."
>
> Alexis, Wainscott, NY

Like the athlete, the massage therapist, who also uses his body to make money, needs a regular regimen of body strengthening and stretching exercises along with aerobic exercise to prepare for the rigors of the work. There are multitudes of disciplines that speak to the specific demands of massage therapy. Over the years, I have explored and practiced many physical and energetic or *qi* (energy) based disciplines. A strengthening and stretching regimen, coupled with qi cultivation or meditation, is a fundamental tool for maintenance of the body, mind, and spirit for a long and healthy career in massage.

> I think my body is starting to tell me that I'm not going to be able to do massage full-time for years and years. I'm hoping that over several years I'll be able to wean myself from five massages, five days a week, to more administrative work and be able to offer more in that area. I'm already experiencing pain in my wrist, in my back, in my arms; my thumb will lock up, and I get headaches. So I have to be more committed to self-maintenance. I'll find myself saying, "Today I can use my left arm or my right arm." It's hard work. I tend to be holistic about it, icing and working on myself.
>
> Tamara, Chicago, IL

Muscle Strengthening

Muscle strengthening is imperative to prevent injury and to ensure that you have the energy to do the last massage at the end of the week with the same focus and vitality as you have for the first of the week. Weightlifting is the conventional form of muscle strengthening, though I have found using elastic bands or cords to be uniquely effective, convenient, and portable. Regardless of the method you use for strength training, it is important to work agonist and antagonist muscle groups evenly by incorporating the breath and working slowly to evenly contract (concentric contraction) and release (eccentric contraction) the muscles, with a strong emphasis on body mechanics. It is a good idea to vary or alternate an exercise regimen to combat boredom and to work muscle groups differently. Recently, I added kettle bells to my strengthening regimen. Kettle bell exercises are good for both an upper- and lower-body workout, but a word of caution with kettle bells, as with all weight exercises: start with light weight to develop good form and body mechanics. The repetitive forward motion of these exercises puts a fair amount of stress on the shoulder joint, a joint that is already stressed by massage work. Strengthening the shoulder joint is a good idea, as long as it is done without overstressing or injuring the joint in the process.

Pilates

Pilates is another strengthening and stretching regimen that is particularly suited to the massage therapist. It focuses on strengthening the core of the body and then working outward, incorporating the breath to strengthen the body through relaxation. One strength of Pilates as a self-care regimen is its focus on the individual needs of the practitioner. The practitioner works to strengthen weak areas and stretch tight areas in an attempt to repattern muscular movement. By working through this model, it can also inform the practitioner not only as a personal self-care tool but also as a diagnostic and rehabilitation tool for using with clients.

Tai Qi

Tai Qi, because of its squatting position and relaxed joints, is a great model for teaching good body mechanics for the beginning therapist. In Tai Qi, all motion originates from the abdomen, thereby lowering the center of gravity. This, combined with the focus on a long, straight spine, is the basis for fundamentally good body mechanics and counteracts the inclination to work from the shoulders in a protracted position. Body alignment in Tai Qi is the first step in what is for some of us a lifelong endeavor to balance and cultivate qi. Aligning the body and the qi to facilitate the work of massage is a discipline well worth the investment, not only to support and prolong our practice of massage but also to support and enrich our lives.

> The most discipline I have is around my meditation practice, so I sit every day. I do Tai Qi on a relatively regular basis. I swim maybe two or three times a week. I'm going to buy a Pilates reformer to strengthen my legs. In my exercise program, I want to make sure I have an open system. The more open I can make myself, the easier it is for me to do my work without hurting myself.
>
> Peggy, Melbourne, FL

Yoga

Yoga is another energy-based discipline that is a wonderful complement to massage. Unlike Tai Qi, which is more dynamic (working through motion), most forms of yoga work through a more static model. There are many different styles of yoga, each with its unique focus. Yoga works to strengthen a group of muscles by working to hold the body in specific positions (asanas) while at the same time stretching the antagonist muscle group. It's a wonderful exploration of yin and yang in the body, contracting and strengthening while simultaneously relaxing and stretching. From a Western perspective, we might define yoga as isometric exercise, where the force of contracting one group of muscles equals the force of stretching its antagonist partners. One thing that all energy-based disciplines share is the focus on the breath. Air and the breath are forms of qi or fuel for the body.

Aerobic Exercise

Aerobic exercise, whether walking, jogging, biking, swimming, or even dance (among many others), with its focus on increasing oxygen intake, is a terrific way to release stress and increase qi production by simply increasing air intake. Swimming is easiest on the joints and is especially good for an upper-body workout but can work the entire body, depending on the stroke. To maintain balance while swimming, try breathing to both sides to keep the neck muscles and cervical spine equally strong and flexible. If you have cervical issues, a snorkel may help. Consider including the backstroke to counteract the repetitive forward action of massage stroking. The breaststroke is also good for the massage therapist, but if done improperly it can exacerbate neck extension and hyperextension problems.

Conversely, biking focuses on the lower body but, depending on the seat and handlebar height, can put a fair amount of stress on the shoulders, wrists, and neck joints. Prolonged hyperextension of the neck along with these other stress points can exacerbate already stressed areas for the massage therapist.

Running or jogging gives the body a good overall workout, but certainly with greater emphasis on the lower body. Elliptical machines simulate running and virtually eliminate the compressive force to the joints of conventional running. Running generally tightens leg, hip, and back muscles, so stretching twenty-four to forty-eight hours after running can ameliorate the tightening effects of a running regimen.

Meditation

Any form of meditation, whether as part of Tai Qi, a yoga practice, or a specific Qi Gong (energy-based meditation) practice, is particularly good for helping us to focus inwardly. Much of our work is extremely physical and extroverted. Finding a meditation practice that helps to counter the physical demands with the ethereal focus of cultivating qi is an invaluable tool for supporting our physical strength and stamina, our mental happiness and well-being, and our spiritual enlightenment.

There are multitudes of body disciplines that are good for cultivating the strength, stamina, and focus required to do massage in a balanced and healthy way. Whenever I advise my students and my clients on exercise and body maintenance, my first suggestion is to find something that they enjoy. Often we discuss where they can find time in their day to exercise or stretch. A self-care discipline will only work if we are likely to do it *regularly*. The rigors and discipline required to maintain the body, the mind, and the spirit are a necessary investment for the success of a massage practice. Our greatest dividend for embracing this discipline is that we are enriched with a more balanced, healthier, and happier life.

Diversity

Varying the strokes you use while giving a massage helps you use different body parts for your work and avoid overtaxing any one body part. Including rest strokes and evaluation strokes between deeper power strokes can help to pace your work in a mindful and healthy way. In the same vein, it is also a good idea to explore different modalities. Adding energetic modalities to your palette of offerings can give overused muscles time to rest and rejuvenate. Consider scheduling more difficult clients with a rest break afterward, and don't forget to consider the pacing and rest intervals in your schedule for a whole week, month, or busy season. This can be a vital tool in managing a more prosperous and healthy career.

> One of the reasons I am doing cranial work is that it doesn't take too much physical strength. I am finding that, physically, by the end of the day, I hurt rather than being just tired. I'm usually okay the next day. I use magnets for my wrist; I swim so my shoulder joints stay mobile. I have learned to use gravity, use good body mechanics, and wait until the tissue responds. I think I'm working smarter so I don't have to work harder.
>
> Peggy, Melbourne, FL

Self-Care Mantras

I have three main phrases I use with my students to remind them of the importance of body mechanics:

1. Keep all joints flexed and relaxed: Throughout the field of massage there are well-known and respected educators who teach the benefit of locking the knee and elbow for added support and strength. I humbly disagree with this approach. I teach from a Tai Qi model, where all joints remain flexed, because an extended and locked joint actually stresses the joint and the surrounding tissue. I believe we actually develop more strength when we allow the joints to stay flexed and the qi (energy) to flow more easily. It is the qi that gives us our strength, not our skeleton. Locked joints, from a martial-arts perspective, actually create vulnerability, because the range of motion for the locked joint is limited and the soft tissue is susceptible to injury or tearing toward the locked direction. When force is added, whether in a healthy way (by leaning) or an unhealthy way (by pressing), the surrounding tissue and joint are unduly stressed. I teach body mechanics with a Tai Qi model because the form builds the strength and stamina necessary for the rigors of massage. Tai Qi is practiced with the spine long and straight, where all motion initiates from the Tanden (Sea of Qi, just below the navel), with the knees (and elbows) flexed so the body remains in a squatted position (as though walking in a low-ceilinged room), thereby lowering the center of gravity and putting the greatest amount of stress on the larger muscles of the legs and not in the lower back or the shoulder girdle. Like the practice of Tai Qi, developing strength and stamina is a process that requires time, discipline, and patience, with the added responsibility of honoring our unique limitations.

2. *Engage the rhomboids:* This is a simple suggestion to avoid the natural tendency to work with our shoulders in a protracted position. Over time this position can lead to thoracic outlet syndrome, among other debilitating conditions. The universe gave us gravity but not good posture. We have to constantly work against gravity to maintain good posture in life as well as at the massage table, consciously choosing to keep ourselves upright and erect. "Engage the rhomboids" is a mantra I suggest to help my students remember not to protract the shoulders while working.

3. *Stay under the ball:* This is another mantra I use to fight the urge to elevate the shoulders in an attempt to achieve greater leverage and strength. This body position is based on a Tai Qi model where the knees and elbows remain flexed, thereby lowering the center of gravity. The therapist consciously depresses the shoulders, keeping the elbows flexed, relaxed, and close to the torso, forcing the therapist to move the (stronger) legs to produce a stroke. The image is one of balancing a large ball on the forearms and creating a stroke that stays "under the ball" rather than elevating the shoulders and elbows "over the ball." This approach often leads to lowering the table to accommodate the slightly squatted body position.

Checklist: Self-Care Quick and Easy

Before a session

Wash hands with warm water
Flexion and rotation: finger, wrist, shoulder
Lightly stretch: forearms, chest, neck, lower back
Standing (vertical) fingertip push-ups

During a session

Breathe
Pay attention to body mechanics
Keep a low center of gravity
Lower the table to fingertip height
Move from the abdomen
Stay close to your work
Move lower body with your strokes
Use body weight for pressure
Tape injured areas for support
Work in layers and sections
Keep all joints flexed and relaxed
Engage the rhomboids
Stay under the ball

After a session

Wash hands and forearms with cold water
Lightly stretch: forearms, chest, neck, lower back
Contrast bathing (alternating ice and heat) for overused body parts:
hands, wrists, elbows
Ice inflamed areas

One thing I know I did when I first started practicing was shuttling back and forth. I would shuttle back and forth between what I was perceiving in the client and what I was perceiving in my own body, so I would constantly monitor how I was using my body and how I was responding to what was going on with them. That has helped me stay in touch with my body mechanics. Another thing that's important is being able to use both sides of the body equally. I consciously chose to use my left arm more. I'm relatively ambidextrous at this point.

Peggy, Melbourne, FL

Paying attention while you're working is an absolute. I don't think I tended to own my body very well at the beginning; I was so focused on the other person. I do a lot of maintenance, self-massage. I start and end my day by really tuning into my own body and stretching and working things out. I do many things like yoga and dance and movement and what I call "downloading" my body after a day's work. A very crucial thing is receiving massage myself. I realized that, along with looking at longevity, I really need to look at something else that isn't as physical to complement, to balance out, so that I can do it for many, many years to come.

Denise, San Francisco, CA

Burnout

Burnout is a very real, potentially career-ending phenomenon common to all health-care professionals. Essentially, burnout is the result of overwork. At our best, with each client we corral the resources and experience of our physical body, the intellect of our mind, and the intuition of our spiritual self to create a unique, cohesive, compassionate, and client-centered massage session. Each client is different and requires summoning our resources differently. The demand to be uniquely effective with each client, session after session, day after day, week after week easily explains the depleting nature of our work and reinforces our need to include rest and rejuvenation in our self-care regimen.

> It has been a struggle to take care of myself well enough. I've gotten burned out. The toll it takes on me is more emotional. I suffer from depression as a result of working so much. I'm trying to give myself plenty of downtime, relaxation time. I do qi movement regularly, every day. That makes the biggest difference, actually. I do some stretching that relaxes my body and my mind.
>
> Tony, Denver, CO

The beginning therapist, eager to build a clientele, finds it difficult to turn clients away. Therapists who take jobs in spas will often do too many massages to boost income, impress their employers, or to consolidate their work hours to allow more time to pursue a private practice or another profession. For the beginning therapist, working in an established massage business has its pros and cons. Having a steady stream of clients is certainly a benefit, though a relentless stream of clients can be debilitating. We need to recognize and honor the limitations of our bodies, minds, and spirits and learn to "just say no." Saying no may be the hardest thing for a young therapist trying to build a practice to utter. We have to consider, though, when we are tired, overworked, and not doing our best work, that besides losing our vitality, we may also lose a client.

> Burnout is not an achy arm or a wrist or thumb or shoulder. Burnout is not physical pain. Burnout is not waking up in the morning and saying, "I'd like to go to the movie instead of going to work." Burnout is getting to the point where even though you've slept eight to ten hours, you need massive amounts of caffeine to make it through the day, and you can never seem to catch up. For days and weeks you obsess on the psycho-emotional things you have heard and learned from your clients and can't seem to clear them out. I don't serve anybody if I am not well. I know that, and it has to be the centerpiece for me and my decision making. So I take extremely good care of myself. I get bodywork, I get chiropractic, I go to the osteopath, I exercise, I train, I take time to read and go to the beach and sit under a tree and meditate, and I spend a lot of time with my daughter and my wife.
>
> Barry, Los Angeles, CA

There are many things you can do to battle fatigue, burnout, and boredom. Besides a regular exercise regimen and meditation practice you can:

Checklist: Avoiding Burnout

1. Take a regular day(s) off
2. Take breaks between clients
3. Get fresh air
4. Take a walk
5. Drink water
6. Stretch
7. Meditate
8. Nap
9. Limit the number of clients / raise your fee
10. Eliminate "draining" clients
11. Follow a heavy day with a light day or a day off
12. Examine your diet
    Eliminate foods with highs and lows: sugar, caffeine, chocolate
    Eat regularly to sustain energy
    Plan ahead
    Carry portable healthy food: Nuts, fruits, vegetables, trail mix, health bars, water
    Eat smaller meals more often
    Eat to eliminate hunger, not to fill up
13. Get regular massage or bodywork
14. Improve your body mechanics
15. Explore different ways of working
    Use different body parts: Forearms, fists, elbows, knees, feet
    Study new techniques: Energetic, physical
16. Develop a referral system
17. Take a relaxing vacation

> When I do massage, I'm always careful. When a client asked me to do specific kinds of work that I didn't do, in the old days I might have tried it and found that I couldn't do it and tried to figure out a way that I could. Now I say, "This is not what I do. I'd be glad to give you the names of people who do this type of work."
>
> Alexis, Wainscott, NY

Because massage requires using our whole being in order to have a sustained, successful, and fulfilling career, we need to examine and work to balance all aspects of our lives—body, mind, and spirit. It is this process that gives us the first-hand experience we need for our work and develops a personal working vocabulary that creates credibility and trust with our clients. Our personal knowledge and discipline becomes an inspiration to them. Listening to our own body's needs is the first step in hearing our clients' needs. In order to trust and rely on our instincts, we have to first develop the sensitivity to hear them. Our bodies are homeostatic organisms, and by nature we are constantly seeking balance. By taking on a profession that requires the use of all our resources, seeking balance needs to be a committed concern. Overwork and overcommitment dulls our senses, our bodies, and our judgment. Recognizing and honoring our limitations in our work as well as our lives is crucial in our path toward balance and success.

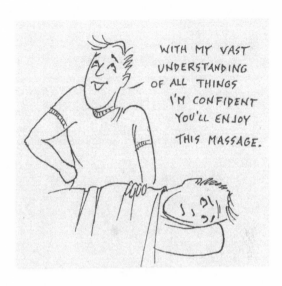

Golden Rule 10

Be informed, not a know-it-all.

Professional and knowledgeable needn't be egotistical.
Listening is better than talking.

Appendix I: History of Massage

There are many varied accounts about the creation and development of massage therapy, spanning several centuries and countless cultures across the globe. The following is a partial timeline that outlines milestones in the development of massage. It is adapted from *The History of Massage* by Robert Noah Calvert and two websites, www.thebodyworker.com/history and www.massagenerd.com/history.

ca. 3000 BC China: *Cong-Fu of the Toa-Tse*, the oldest known book about massage, is written. (It remains unknown in the West until it is translated into French in the 1700s.)

2760 BC China: The earliest surviving text on traditional Chinese medicine, the Yellow Emperor's *Inner Canon* or *Huangdi Neijing Suwen*, discusses therapeutic touch.

ca. 2500 BC Egypt: Egyptians create their form of reflexology.

ca. 1800 BC India: Classic Ayurvedic texts, which view health as an integral part of spiritual life, include massage techniques.

ca. 1700 BC China: Tui Na, a form of Chinese manipulative therapy, dates back to the Shang dynasty.

776 BC Greece: In the Olympic Games, athletes are massaged prior to their events.

ca. 500 BC Greece: Herodicus is the first person to combine sports with medicine. Considered to be the founder of what we now call sports medicine, he prescribes specific gymnastic exercises for healing.

ca. 500 BC Thailand: Thai massage is created combining traditions and techniques from Ayurvedic medicine, Buddhist spiritual practice, Chinese medicine and yoga, and indigenous healing practices. It is used to treat disease and disharmony of physical, emotional, and spiritual origins. Nuad Bo Rarn is the traditional medical massage.

460–380 BC Greece: Hippocrates, a student of Herodicus, uses friction to treat sprains and dislocations. He believes that disease results from natural causes and that the body has the power to heal itself, and he writes the code of ethics that we know as the Hippocratic Oath.

100–44 BC Rome: Julius Caesar receives massage therapy to relieve his neuralgia and epileptic seizures.

ca. 50 AD Rome: Aulus Cornelius Celsus, an encyclopedist, writes *De Medicina*, a portion of a larger medical encyclopedia that includes information on massage, diet, pharmacy, and surgery. It is considered one of the best sources of medical knowledge in the Roman world.

ca. 100 AD China: The earliest texts describing Qi Gong date to the first or second century, and the first schools of massage appear.

130–201 AD Rome: Galen, a disciple of Hippocrates and physician to gladiators and emperors, writes multiple medical texts, his most famous a work on anatomy. Another, *Hygiene,* reveals his respect for massage. In the chapter entitled "Morning and Evening Massage," he describes in detail massage strokes and their physiological benefits.

5th–15th centuries AD Europe: Exercise and massage, integral parts of life in the Roman Empire, virtually disappear after the fall of the Empire. The new dominant religion, Christianity, deemphasizes the human body in favor of the salvation of the soul.

ca. 600 AD Japan: Shiatsu, or acupressure, is developed.

980–1037 Baghdad: Avicenna, the chief physician at the Baghdad hospital, writes medicinal texts that include sections on techniques and effects of massage.

1363 France: Guy de Chauliac, physician to three popes, writes *Chirurgia magna*, the standard text on surgery for the next two centuries, mentioning bodywork as an adjunct to surgery.

1510–1590 Paris: Ambrose Paré, the renowned physician to four French kings who is considered one of the fathers of surgery, is a strong advocate of mechanical treatments, including exercise and massage.

1514–1564 Italy: Andreas Vesalius, a professor at the University of Padua, creates the first major studies of human anatomy, which become an essential part of medical and massage studies.

1569 Italy: Girolamo Mercuriali writes the first sports medicine book, *De Gymnastica,* with passages on exercise and manual therapies.

ca. 1600 London: Sir Francis Bacon observes that massage has benefits enhancing circulation.

1660–1742 Halle, Germany: Friedrich Hoffman publishes *Dissertationes Physico-Medicae.* With a chapter describing movement as the best medicine for the body, he establishes a model for medical gymnastics.

1742–1823 London: English surgeon John Grosvenor practices healing with the hands and is known especially for his treatment of stiff and diseased joints by friction.

1776–1837 Sweden: Per Henrik Ling, a fencing master and gymnast, combines earlier disparate knowledge of medical gymnastics into a systematized method, based on anatomy and physiology, that applies exercise and gymnastics to treat specific disorders as well as to maintain health. His system of soft tissue techniques includes active, active-passive, and passive manipulation. The passive manipulations in his system are the beginnings of what will later become the basic strokes of Swedish massage, and many people now credit him as the father of Swedish massage.

ca. 1800 Japan: Philosopher and Christian seminary educator Dr. Mikao Usui is the founder of the spiritual practice of Reiki.

1825 Philadelphia: Bache Franklin, MD, a great-grandson of Benjamin Franklin, translates Morand's *Memoir on Acupuncture* from the French, and it becomes the first treatise on acupuncture available in America.

1828–1917 United States: American osteopathic medicine is established by Andrew Taylor Still, who also founds the American School of

Osteopathy (now A. T. Still University) in Kirksville, Missouri, in 1892.

1839–1909 Holland: Physician Johann Georg Mezger is considered by some the more likely candidate for the title of "the father of Swedish Massage," for simplifying the passive movements of Ling's medical gymnastic system. He adopts the French terms *effleurage, petrissage, friction,* and *tapotement* for the techniques that are generally used to define Swedish massage.

1851 Brighton, England: Mathias Roth, an orthopedic surgeon, homeopath, and strong advocate of Ling's Swedish movement system, writes *The Prevention and Cure of Many Diseases by Movements.* The medical establishment of the time finds his views suspect, whereas the *British Journal of Homeopathy* reviews it enthusiastically.

1856 England: Charles Fayette Taylor and George Herbert Taylor (who also studied in Sweden) study with Roth in England and bring massage to the United States. George Taylor develops a system of exercise therapy.

1866 London: Walter Johnson writes *The Anatriptic Art: A History of the Art Termed Anatriptic by Hippocrates, Tripsis by Galen, Frictio by Celsus, Manipulation by Beveridge and Medical Rubbing in Ordinary Language.* He not only defines the terms used to describe massage throughout history, but his comprehensive text provides case histories where symptoms are defined, diagnosis and treatments are applied, and the results are detailed.

1879 Boston: Douglas Graham describes the Hawaiian massage modality Lomi lomi and writes a history of massage.

1884 Paris: Jean-Martin Charcot, the father of neurology (and teacher of Sigmund Freud, among others) believes that French doctors should use massage more.

1887 London: Dr. William Murrell writes *Massage as a Mode of Treatment,* where he further defines massage as a medical treatment modality, separating it from massage of "the baths." His work was perhaps the first to espouse the benefits of massage from an experimental, scientific viewpoint. He believes that massage practitioners must have specialized training.

1887 New York: George H. Taylor, MD, publishes *Massage: Principles and Practice of Remedial Treatment by Imparted Motion* and *Health by Exercise: The Movement Cure.* He describes active and passive massage techniques, echoing Per Henrik Ling's method of medical gymnastics.

1888 Sweden: Dr. Emil Kleen writes *Handbook of Massage,* in which he is critical of Ling's lack of scientific training. Kleen draws a distinction between medical gymnastic movements, orthopaedic treatments, and massage and countenances the employment of all three in combination.

1889 Philadelphia: Hartvig (Harvey) Nissen writes *A Manual of Instruction for Giving Swedish Movement and Massage Treatment.* He considers massage, though an adjunct of medical gymnastics, to be a separate form of treatment. He outlines specific cases to highlight the work's efficacy and defines the concept of contraindications for the use of massage.

1894 England: The Society of Trained Masseuses establishes the formal study of massage, along with prerequisites for education and criteria for the recognition of massage schools.

1895 Battle Creek, Michigan: John Harvey Kellogg, chief medical officer of the Battle Creek Sanitarium, renowned for its holistic medical techniques, publishes *The Art of Massage: A Practical Manual for the Nurse, the Student, and the Practitioner.* He espouses massage and systematic rubbing and manipulation as one of the oldest techniques for relieving the body of infirmities. He commends Ling's systematic medical gymnastics. He is a strong advocate of vegetarianism, develops a highly successful brand of corn flakes, and patents a process for making peanut butter. A bitter feud erupts with his brother over the recipe for their breakfast cereal (his brother wants to add sugar) that leads to a split and the formation of two separate companies, the Kellogg Co. and the Battle Creek Food Co.

1897 Boston: Axel V. Grafstrom, MD, publishes *A Text-book of Mechano-Therapy (Massage and Medical Gymnastics)* based on the system employed by the Royal Gymnastic Central Institute in Stockholm, Sweden. The text distinguishes between medical gymnastic movements (active and passive range of motion, with and without resistance) and passive massage techniques. It includes detailed descriptions of massage strokes and their applications for specific conditions and diseases.

1899 London: Sir William Bennett starts a massage department at St. George's Hospital and publishes *Lectures on the Use of Massage* in 1910.

ca. 1900 England: Australian actor F. Matthias Alexander develops the Alexander Technique, focusing on body coordination and awareness to improve freedom and efficiency of movement.

1901 United States: Benedict Lust develops naturopathy, based on the idea that the body can heal itself. He opens the American School of Naturopathy in New York City and launches the Naturopathic Society of America in 1902.

1902 United States: Douglas Graham publishes *Manual Therapeutics: A Treatise on Massage.* He describes the use of massage by different cultures, including the Chinese, the Egyptians, and the Greeks, as well as its use in healing rituals by the Navajo Indians, in the laying on of hands by Christians, and by the Hawaiians in a form of massage called Lomi lomi.

1904 New York City: The Swedish Gymnastic Institute is founded by Captain Theodore Melander, a graduate of the Swedish Royal Military Academy. It later becomes the Swedish Institute (1916), the largest massage school in the country.

1907 England: Edgar Ferdinand Cyriax, a physiotherapist

of Swedish origin, uses Ling's Swedish Movement Cure and Mechanotherapeutics.

1911 England: Louisa Despard, an Irish nurse, writes *The Book of Massage and Remedial Gymnastics,* which becomes widely used for training in English hospitals. The largest text of its kind for the time, it contained 395 pictures and plates and 450 pages of text divided into two sections, the first part devoted to anatomy and physiology and the second to massage theory and application.

1913 United States: William Fitzgerald, MD, the father of modern reflexology, rediscovers reflexology and calls it Zone Therapy.

1916 New York: The Swedish Institute of Physiotherapy, formerly the Swedish Gymnastic Institute, becomes the first massage training institute in the United States.

1921 Boston: Mary McMillan, RN, writes *Massage and Therapeutic Exercise.* Out of the ravages of World War I and the polio epidemic emerges the need for "reconstruction aides," and so the field of physical therapy is born. In her book, McMillan acknowledges the genesis of a new field of study and defines four distinct branches: massage, therapeutic exercise, electrotherapy, and hydrotherapy. She espouses the importance of linking the various branches of treatment "for the most beneficial results." She later becomes director of physiotherapy at Harvard Medical School and the founder of the American Physical Therapy Association.

1923 Germany: Albert Hoffa writes *Technike der Massage,* which describes many of the techniques currently in use today.

1925 United States: Joseph Pilates emigrates from Germany and continues to develop the Pilates method, a set of exercises that strengthen the core of the body. He opens a studio in New York and goes on to write several books, including *Return to Life through Contrology* and *Your Health.*

1927 New York: The first professional massage association, the New York State Society of Medical Massage Therapists, is formed.

ca. 1930 England: Stanley Leif and Boris Chaitow, cousins trained in osteopathy and naturopathy, create neuromuscular therapy, a manual treatment protocol targeting soft tissue injuries and chronic pain dysfunctions.

1932 Maryland: Kathryn Jensen, RN, director of physical therapy instruction at Washington Sanitarium and Hospital, writes *Fundamentals in Massage for Students of Nursing*. She broaches the idea that massage need not be the exclusive realm of the medical field but should be put into the hands of specialists.

1933 St. Louis, Missouri: As the requirements for training in massage are increased, Maude Rawlins, MD, writes *A Textbook of Massage for Nurses and Beginners*.

1934 Vienna: Wilhelm Reich, an Austrian psychoanalyst and student of Freud's, brings body awareness into psychiatry, using somatic techniques to dissolve muscular "armor." Bioenergetics, created by Alexander Lowen, later emerges from Reich's work.

1936 Paris: Emil Voder, a Danish physiologist who has studied the lymphatic system in depth, introduces the Voder system of manual lymph drainage.

1937 France: Rene-Maurice Gattefosse, a chemist studying essential oils, begins his research into the healing powers of essential oils after burning his hand badly in his laboratory and immersing it in lavender oil. He is impressed by how quickly the burn heals, publishes a book about the antimicrobial effects of the oils, and coins the word aromatherapy.

1939 United States: The Florida State Massage Therapy Association is organized, and in 1943 Florida becomes the first state to enact standards for regulating massage training and practice.

1940 England: Osteopath James Cyriax, the son of Edgar Cyriax, creates the Cyriax System of orthopedic medicine, which utilizes deep transverse friction.

1940 Japan: Tokujiro Namikoshi establishes the Japan Shiatsu College. One of his students, Tadashi Izawa, creates meridian shiatsu, and another, Shizuto Masunaga, creates Zen shiatsu.

1940 Michigan: The Battle Creek Company manufactures the first lightweight, portable massage table, made of aluminum.

1943 Illinois: The Chicago American Association of Masseurs and Masseuses is formed. Later it becomes the American Massage Therapy Association, the first nationwide professional association for the industry.

1952 New York: Janet Travell, MD, researches trigger points and their relationship to myofascial pain syndrome. Later, as John F. Kennedy's personal physician, she treats his chronic back pain during his time in the Senate and in the White House, becoming the first woman to be appointed personal physician to a sitting president.

1956 California: Margaret Knott and Dorothy Vass write a book called *Proprioceptive Neuromuscular Facilitation,* based on their teaching and the work of their mentor, Herman Kabat, a doctor who, with Henry J. Kaiser, founded the Kabat-Kaiser Institute in California to study neuromuscular disorders.

ca. 1960 Pennsylvania: John Barnes, a physical therapist, develops myofascial release therapy. He publishes *Myofascial Release: The Search for Excellence* in 1990.

1962 Big Sur, California: The Esalen Institute is founded as a center to explore human potential and becomes known for its integration of Eastern and Western philosophies. Philosophers, psychologists, artists, and religious thinkers—including Ida Rolf (*Rolfing: The Integration of Human Structures*), Deane Juhan (*Job's Body*), and Bernie Gunther (*Sense*

Relaxation, Energy Ecstasy, Neo-Tantra, Dying for Enlightenment)—
study and train others at Esalen.

1964 Illinois: Gertrude Beard, RN, PT, and Elizabeth C. Wood publish
their classic textbook *Massage: Principles and Techniques.*

1964 Michigan: Chiropractor George J. Goodheart Jr. develops applied
kinesiology. The International College of Applied Kinesiology is founded
in 1975 to provide instruction based on Goodheart's research.

1972 Tel Aviv: Physicist Moshé Feldenkrais develops the Feldenkrais
Method, designed to improve overall body function by increasing
self-awareness through movement. He publishes *Awareness Through
Movement,* a follow-up to his 1949 publication, *Body and Mature
Behavior.*

1972 Big Sur, California: George Downing publishes a pioneering
compendium, *The Massage Book,* with illustrations by Anne Kent Rush,
still a classic text used around the world.

1973 Massachusetts: Zero Balancing, a hands-on body/mind system, is
developed by osteopath and acupuncturist Dr. Fritz Smith. It integrates
Eastern and Western medical philosophies, teaching how to align body
energy with the body's physical structure.

1977 Kennewick, Washington: Ruth E. Williams publishes *The Road
to Radiant Health*, a massage textbook used in schools throughout the
country.

1978 California: Joseph Heller, a student of Ida Rolf, starts
Hellerwork, incorporating movement education and body-centered
human development processes for a body, mind, spirit approach to
bodywork.

1978 Buckley, Washington: Soma Neuromuscular Integration (Soma
Bodywork) is developed by Bill Williams, PhD, another student of
Ida Rolf. His work expands the focus of Rolf's work to incorporate

psychology and energy into a body-mind-spirit model for health and healing.

ca. 1980 California: Watsu (Water shiatsu) is developed by Harold Dull, a student of Harbin School of Shiatsu and Massage, whose director Shizuto Masunaga also created Zen shiatsu.

1983 United States: Janet Travell (with David Simons) publishes the two-volume text *Myofascial Pain and Dysfunction: The Trigger Point Manual.*

ca. 1990 San Francisco: David Palmer is credited as the "father of chair massage" for the significant role he plays in the growth of on-site massage. He is the founder of TouchPro Institute, a professional organization that provides training for chair massage.

1991 Miami: The Touch Research Institute, the first center in the world devoted to the study of touch and its application in science and medicine, is established by Tiffany Field, PhD.

1991 New York: The state legislature changes the title of a massage professional to Massage Therapist. Licensure confers the title Licensed Massage Therapist.

1992 United States: The National Certification Board for Therapeutic Massage and Bodywork (NCBTMB) is established and begins the process to nationally regulate and certify massage in the United States.

1992 Atlanta: To balance the shift toward technologically oriented care, Andy Bernay-Roman, RN, founds the National Association of Nurse Massage Therapists to bring a more holistic approach to health care.

1993 China: Sun Chengnan publishes *Chinese Bodywork, A Complete Manual of Chinese Therapeutic Massage.* The book reflects the teachings of the Shandong school and covers massage methods, theory, and applications. It includes modern techniques of Chinese Tui Na to treat chronic disease.

1995 Lapeer, Michigan: Sandy Fritz publishes the first edition of her best-selling textbook, *Mosby's Fundamentals of Therapeutic Massage.*

1996 India: Harish Johari, a scholar, author, artist, and composer, publishes *Ayurvedic Massage*, about an Eastern form of bodywork that focuses on balancing the body's energy, not unlike shiatsu.

Appendix II: Massage Modalities

Massage Modalities	
Acupressure: see Shiatsu	
Alexander Technique	Founded by F. Mathias Alexander, this technique focuses on balancing posture and movement efficiently by relearning patterns of movement through simple and repetitive exercises like standing, sitting, and walking.
Anma	Anma means to press (An) and to rub (Ma). One of the oldest forms of bodywork, it developed in China 5,000 years ago from roots in ancient India, Korea, and Japan. It has influenced other forms of massage such as shiatsu, Tui Na, and even Swedish massage. It works to stimulate the skin and specific points, or tsubos, in order to release tension and balance the flow of energy in the body.
Applied Kinesiology	Established in 1964 by George Goodheart, this chiropractic diagnostic method uses manual muscle-strength testing for medical diagnosis of corresponding organs and systems. It attempts an integrated, interdisciplinary approach to health care, including manual manipulations and nutritional supplements.
Aromatherapy	Aromatherapy is the practice of using volatile plant oils, including essential oils, for psychological and physical well-being. It is used by practitioners including massage therapists, chiropractors, nurses, and doctors.
Ayurvedic Massage	A 3,000-year-old practice that originated in India. Using the hands and the feet, the therapist works on Marma pressure points—areas where flesh, veins, arteries, tendons, bones, and joints meet—in order to protect, activate, and balance prana (energy). The 107 Marma points are manipulated to stimulate and treat the internal organs in order to cure or control disease.

Bindegewebmassage or Connective Tissue Massage	Developed in 1929 by Elizabeth Dicke in Germany, Bindegewebmassage is similar in theory to shiatsu and acupuncture. Light strokes are applied to the skin, targeting the superficial fascia with the overall intention of affecting the underlying organs and tissue to promote health and healing.
Craniosacral Therapy	Craniosacral therapy, created by Dr. John Upledger, uses light manipulation of the skull and other parts of the body in order to assess and affect the rhythmic flow of the cerebral spinal fluid that surrounds the brain and spinal cord to treat a myriad of ailments including chronic pain, migraines, TMJ, depression, and tinnitus.
Cyriax Method	Created in the 1920s by Dr. James Cyriax, an English internist and orthopedic surgeon who developed a series of simple clinical exams to diagnose soft tissue musculoskeletal lesions. His work produced a systematic set of clinical exams for each joint and a treatment system for the soft tissue lesions around them. He coined the term orthopedic medicine.
Deep Tissue Massage	A form of Swedish massage that attempts to assess specific muscular and fascial imbalances and employs deep massage strokes to improve posture, function, and performance and relieve pain.
Feldenkrais Method	Introduced Dr. Moshé Feldenkrais, who used movement and body manipulations to bring an active awareness to unconscious patterns of movement in order to reduce pain and discomfort and promote muscular efficiency.
Lomi lomi	A Hawaiian massage modality with a spiritual influence, Lomi lomi employs long, broad strokes using the forearms and hands to perform deep tissue techniques.

Lymphatic Drainage	Lymphatic drainage, created by Emil Voder, is an extremely light and gentle form of massage that targets the lymphatic system in order to affect lymph flow. It is used specifically to reduce swelling and edema, especially after surgery where lymph nodes and vessels are removed or damaged.
Myofascial Release	Myofascial release targets the fascia and connective tissue in the body using long, deep, and generally slow strokes in order to relieve chronic pain and improve posture and muscular function.
Neuromuscular Therapy	Neuromuscular therapy uses static pressure on myofascial trigger points to affect the central nervous system, relieve pain, and restore range of motion and good posture. NMT addresses five elements that cause pain and dysfunction: ischemia, trigger points, nerve compression or entrapment, postural distortion, and biomechanical dysfunction.
Polarity Therapy	Developed by Dr. Randolph Stone, polarity therapy is comprehensive in its scope, involving energy-based bodywork, diet, exercise, and self-awareness. There are three types of energy fields in the human body that run north-south, east-west and in spiral currents that start at the navel and expand outward. Polarity therapy seeks to release blockages in these fields.
Reflexology or Zone Therapy	This therapy uses pressure on reflex zones in the feet, hands, and ears that correspond to different organs and areas of the body to relieve stress and restore function. Generally the feet are the primary area of treatment and pressure is applied without the use of lotions or oils.

Reiki	Reiki, created by Mikau Usui, is an energy-based modality where the practitioner places her hands over the client's body in an attempt to balance the energy of the chakras. There are two main practices, traditional Reiki and Western Reiki. The work is done clothed without lotions or oil, and there are three levels or degrees of practice. At the first level, the practitioner can heal himself and others; at the second level, the practitioner can heal others at a distance; and at the masters/teacher level, the practitioner can teach and also work with animals and plants.
Rolfing (Structural Integration)	Created by Ida P. Rolf in the 1940s and 1950s, this practice targets the fascia or connective tissue that is responsible for the overall structure and shape of the body. Postural distortions, injury, and scar tissue can affect the function of the fascia and cause stiffness, pain, or decreased range of motion. Through a ten-part series of deep tissue techniques, Rolfing aims to release tension in the fascia, thereby restoring function and posture and relieving pain.
Shiatsu (acupressure)	Traditionally performed clothed on a mat on the floor. The practitioner uses stretching and compression techniques along meridian lines and acupuncture points to balance energy or qi in the body. The practice uses a comprehensive body-mind-spirit approach to health and healing.
Sports Massage	Sports massage is a form of Swedish massage initially designed for athletes to prepare for and recover from sporting events and training sessions. There are four types of sports massage: pre-event, post-event, restorative, and rehabilitative. Generally sports massage targets a specific area of the body in order to enhance performance.

Swedish Massage	Swedish massage is defined by five basic strokes: effleurage, pettrisage, vibration, tapotment, and friction. By manipulating the skin, muscles, and connective tissues of the body, it affects all the systems of the body, promoting general health, relaxation, and well-being.
Thai Massage	Thai massage is believed to have been developed more than 2,500 years ago in India by Jivaka Kumar Bhaccha, "the father doctor" and physician to the Buddha. It was imported to Thailand and influenced by Ayurvedic and traditional Chinese medicine. It is similar to shiatsu, with its focus on the energetic body, mind, and spirit, and is traditionally done on mats on the floor. There are four aspects to the work—massage, diet, spiritual practice, and herbal medicine.
Therapeutic Touch	Therapeutic touch is a misnomer, because the therapist rarely touches the client's body. It is a form of energy work where the therapist moves his or her hands over the client, trying to balance the flow of qi. The intent is to restore the client's energy field to a state of balance or harmony, making it possible for the body to heal itself.
Trager	Developed in the 1920s by Milton Trager, Trager work consists of deep, hands-on work, including fluid, gentle, rocking movements, to produce positive sensory feelings that are then fed back into the central nervous system. The motion in the muscles and joints result in a feeling of lightness and increased flexibility. Simple exercises called mentastics are prescribed to help the client recreate the sensory feelings.

Trigger Point Massage	Janet Travell is recognized as the leading pioneer in developing trigger point therapy. The medical establishment treats trigger points in a multitude of ways, from needling them to injecting them with local anesthetics, steroids, or even botulinum toxin, in order to alleviate symptoms. In the field of massage there are also multiple approaches for treating trigger points. Direct pressure accompanied by different stretching techniques like active isolated stretching techniques and proprioceptive neuromuscular facilitation techniques are employed to reduce pain and improve function.
Tui Na	Tui Na literally translates to "pushing" and "grasping." This ancient hands-on practice has its roots in another therapeutic massage technique called Anmo, which means "pressing" and "rubbing." In ancient China, medical practices were divided into internal and external treatments. Tui Na was one of the external methods used to treat musculoskeletal disorders and stress-related disorders as well as digestive, respiratory, and reproductive ailments. The practitioner employs brushing, kneading, rolling, pressing, and rubbing techniques to affect the qi and blood in the body to try to restore balance and harmony.
Watsu	Watsu, created by Harold Dull, is a form of Zen shiatsu performed in a heated pool, allowing the work to access deeper layers of energetic and emotional relaxation and release. With buoyancy reducing the impact of gravity, the spine, muscles, and joints are more easily stretched, manipulated, and freed. The session alternates between static floating to dance-like choreography while being supported and cradled in the water.

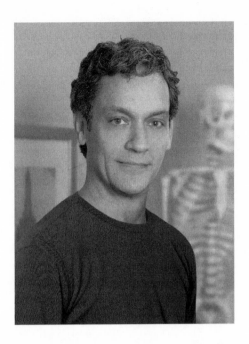

Michael Alicia began a private massage practice after receiving his certification from the Swedish Institute in 1992. He owns and operates Massage Space NYC, which offers bodywork and advanced massage training classes and provides teachers with a forum for developing new workshops. Michael teaches at his studio and the Swedish Institute, and is an adjunct professor at the Therapeutic Massage Training Institute in Charlotte, North Carolina.

Michael's original workshops include: "The Complete Neck Series," "The Money Stroke," "Better Body Mechanics," "Spa Shiatsu," and "Table Thai." The DVD based on his ever-popular workshop *The Stretching Process* is available for purchase online.

More information about Michael and Massage Space NYC is available at www.massagespacenyc.com.

Photo by Rick Schwab
www.rickschwab.net